Secrets
of Successful
Program Design

A How-To Guide
for Busy Fitness Professionals

Secrets of Successful Program Design

A How-To Guide
for Busy Fitness Professionals

Alwyn Cosgrove, CSCS
Craig Rasmussen, CSCS

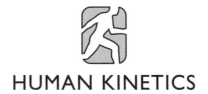

HUMAN KINETICS

Library of Congress Cataloging-in-Publication Data

Names: Cosgrove, Alwyn, author. | Rasmussen, Craig, author.
Title: Secrets of successful program design : a how-to guide for busy
    fitness professionals / Alwyn Cosgrove, Craig Rasmussen.
Description: Champaign, IL : Human Kinetics, 2021.
Identifiers: LCCN 2020007650 (print) | LCCN 2020007651 (ebook) | ISBN
    9781492593225 (paperback) | ISBN 9781492593232 (epub) | ISBN
    9781492593249 (pdf)
Subjects: LCSH: Physical education and training. | Exercise.
Classification: LCC GV711.5 .C67 2021 (print) | LCC GV711.5 (ebook) | DDC
    613.7/1--dc23
LC record available at https://lccn.loc.gov/2020007650
LC ebook record available at https://lccn.loc.gov/2020007651
ISBN: 978-1-4925-9322-5 (print)

This publication is written and published to provide accurate and authoritative information relevant to the subject matter presented. It is published and sold with the understanding that the author and publisher are not engaged in rendering legal, medical, or other professional services by reason of their authorship or publication of this work. If medical or other expert assistance is required, the services of a competent professional person should be sought.

The web addresses cited in this text were current as of March 2020, unless otherwise noted.

Acquisitions Editor: Michael Mejia; **Developmental Editor:** Laura Pulliam; **Managing Editor:** Miranda K. Baur; **Copyeditor:** Lisa Himes; **Permissions Manager:** Martha Gullo; **Graphic Designers:** Whitney Milburn and Dawn Sills; **Cover Designer:** Keri Evans; **Cover Design Specialist:** Susan Rothermel Allen; **Photograph (cover):** jacoblund/iStock/Getty Images; **Photographs (interior):** © Human Kinetics, unless otherwise noted; **Photo Production Specialist:** Amy Rose; **Photo Production Manager:** Jason Allen; **Senior Art Manager:** Kelly Hendren; **Illustrations:** © Human Kinetics; **Printer:** Sheridan Books

We thank Results Fitness in Santa Clarita, CA, for assistance in providing the location for the photo shoot for this book.

Human Kinetics books are available at special discounts for bulk purchase. Special editions or book excerpts can also be created to specification. For details, contact the Special Sales Manager at Human Kinetics.

Printed in the United States of America   10 9 8 7 6 5 4 3 2 1

The paper in this book is certified under a sustainable forestry program.

Human Kinetics
1607 N. Market Street
Champaign, IL 61820
USA

United States and International
Website: **US.HumanKinetics.com**
Email: info@hkusa.com
Phone: 1-800-747-4457

Canada
Website: **Canada.HumanKinetics.com**
Email: info@hkcanada.com

E7916

Tell us what you think!
Human Kinetics would love to hear what we can do to improve the customer experience. Use this QR code to take our brief survey.

This is for all of our colleagues and mentors
who have educated us over so many years.
Thank you for all that you have taught us.

Contents

PART III   Evaluation and Progression

Preface

At our gym, Results Fitness, we are known for writing programs, not just workouts. But what do we mean by this? What is the difference between a program and a workout?

A *program* is an overall training plan that is written based on a particular goal—*plan* and *goal* being the operative words. A single workout (or training session) is a part of this plan, and the structured sequencing of multiple workouts, or daily training sessions is a portion of programming. A *workout* is simply what you do on any given training day. Looked at by itself, without respect to the rest of the overall plan, the individual workout doesn't amount to much.

Periodization is a term that has varying definitions, but most would agree that it means using structured planning and manipulation of training variables to achieve a desired training response over a certain time period.

When creating a program, we always look at the big picture first, figuring out the client's goals, and then estimating how long it will take to reach them. From there, we create an overall long-term periodization plan, or macrocycle. This plan can cover a minimum of 8 to 12 weeks for specific short-term goals, but it can also encompass 16 weeks up to a year. Once we have determined the time frame, we can get more specific and divide the schedule into mesocycles, which are typically 4- to 6-week blocks of time. From there, we add increasingly detailed plans for specific training weeks, or microcycles. Finally, we divide it even further and design each individual training day (or workout), for which we choose exercises, tempos, and rest periods.

We begin with the big picture in mind, then break things down to the individual workout level. Novice coaches and trainers will typically start in the opposite manner, with a mentality of "What exercise am I going to do today?" They will then design a random workout for a particular day using their favorite exercise without regard for the long-term plan. This is an ineffective approach; we want to attain the desired results by executing a properly considered plan and not achieve these results as a possible side effect from a string of random workouts.

As a busy fitness professional, you will soon realize that programming for clients will take up a large portion of your time and energy—especially if you are trying to "cook from scratch" each time you create a training program. You will quickly learn that the lack of a programming system will cause you to repeat mistakes. *Hint:* You need a recipe. So, the big question is "How do you create a sound programming system?" Rest assured, you are in the correct place.

SYSTEM is an acronym that we talk about at our gym, Results Fitness. What does it stand for? There are several versions, but the one we like best is this: **S**ave **Y**ourself **S**ubstantial **T**ime, **E**nergy, and **M**oney. Mark Verstegen, founder of EXOS (a health and human performance company widely renowned for their systems-based approach), has also stated that one of the most important aspects of using systems is to help us avoid making repeated mistakes. Mistakes are always going to happen. They are a big part of how we learn, but we want to avoid continually repeating the same mistakes, because they will become massive problems for us moving forward.

Successful businesses rely upon the ability to implement and execute systems. In some of his lectures about systems, Alwyn has mentioned how a McDonald's Big Mac is the same in Los Angeles as it is in China. You can trust that a Big Mac will be the same wherever you are because they make it the same way. I'm sure that you're thinking that you can get a better hamburger somewhere else, but the point isn't about the quality of the hamburger—it is the fact that McDonald's can faithfully reproduce a desired result because they use a system; they don't try to reinvent the Big Mac with each and every one they make. "Winging it" is a recipe for disaster; following a system is a recipe for success. For this reason, fitness programming must also be system based.

The majority of clients seek help from fitness coaches for one of three primary reasons:

1. They want to look better (lose fat or gain muscle).
2. They want to perform better in a physical pursuit or sporting activity.
3. They want to improve how they feel and move.

That is it! I know this may seem simple, but the simplicity is intentional. Things get more complex when we address highly specific goals, but when we sit down with a client in their initial strategy session, we immediately know that their programming is going to fall into one of those three categories.

If we know this at the outset, we can start to create appropriate programming templates that will help a client reach specific training goals. If we determine that the age and training goals of two different clients are similar, the parameters of their programs will be—and should be—more similar than different, because the two starting points are in the same general area. We can establish a plan in advance, in terms of variables such as reps, sets, tempos, rest periods, and movement patterns on the macro-, meso-, and micro-levels if we are aware of the similarities. This is where templates, or frameworks, come into play because we can outline an exercise selection plan ahead of time. Templates simply provide a premade plan and then allow for small (or large) adjustments based on additional individual information.

Creating a seemingly unique program from scratch for every new client is an unwise decision in terms of time efficiency. Making something different just for the sake of being different is, in fact, bad programming.

What do I mean by that? Let's use an example of two twins (twin A and twin B) who each want to lose 20 pounds (9 kg) of fat and have never done any form of resistance training. I determine that goblet squats would be the best exercise for both of them, but since they are training together and I told them that I would write individualized programs for each of them, I assign goblet squats to twin A and overhead squats to twin B so the programs appear different. But now I may have made twin B's program less effective by presenting an exercise that is too advanced and that may not deliver the results that the goblet squat could, just for the sake of making their programs appear different. This was a misguided reason (there are good reasons at times) because it will compromise potential results. If the exercise choice, rep ranges, and number of sets is the same for two similar clients with similar goals, it is because it is the best choice for both of them right now; thus their training program is still individualized even though the programs may be the same.

There are four main steps to program design:

1. Determine our goal.
2. Determine our starting point (training status).
3. Determine our time frame.
4. Plan backward and execute forward.

If programming is systemized, step four (the planning process) is preset; we can save a lot of time and energy, because most of the major decisions have been made in advance based on goals and training status. We will examine these four steps in greater detail later.

This book presents several real-world plans that have been used to attain specific results and that will give you the skills you need to take your own programming to the next level through the use of a system-based approach. Let's face facts: We're time-constrained fitness professionals, and it is often logistically impossible to spend two to three hours writing an individualized program for every client. It is what we like to call "logistically undesirable." The good news is that this logistically undesirable approach is also not as effective at delivering results as the systemized approach.

We are going to give you a peek behind the curtain and share how we design world-class programs that deliver consistent results to our real-world clientele of varying ages and goals.

In the pages ahead you will find several predesigned plans for your use as well as tools to assess and screen your client's incoming movement qualities with respect to training age. We will explore exercise progressions, regressions, and staple movement patterns based on your client's current state of training preparedness. This is not theoretical made-up programming; this is field-tested, tried and true programming that has been developed and used in our gym-lab for almost two decades.

Acknowledgments

Alwyn: This book is dedicated to the members and team members of Results Fitness. Thank you for the last twenty years.

Craig: I attended a Perform Better event several years ago where performance coach Martin Rooney gave a presentation on the impact of the coach. As part of his talk, he stated that one of the biggest impacts of a coach is that they believe in you more than you believe in yourself. This resonated strongly with me and got me thinking back to the coaches that believed in me throughout my life. As a youth, I struggled with being self-conscience and I had some real issues with shyness. In my late teens and early twenties, I discovered weight training and was "bitten by the iron bug" when I saw what it could do for me and my self-confidence. Over the years I have had several coaches and mentors believe in me more than I believed in myself. There are so many to thank but I only have space to thank a few.

To Randy Rick, my freshman basketball coach. You probably don't know this but taking those three hours out of your day in 1984 to teach me how to shoot a jump shot more than likely put me on the coaching path and taught me so much about how the details matter.

To John Christy, my first strength coach and first mentor in the field of coaching. You were the first to teach me what coaching was all about and how to be a professional in this field. You were the ultimate manifestation of believing in someone more than they believed in themselves. You never placed limiting beliefs on me, or any of your coaching charges. You inspired me to think big and gave me the gift of true self-confidence manifested in the iron. I am forever thankful to have had you and your family in my life. I wish you were still here, my friend, so that I could talk shop with you and tell you about all the wonderful people and coaches I have met, the things that I have learned from them, and the experiences that I have had over the past 11 years since your untimely passing. I miss you greatly.

To Alwyn and Rachel Cosgrove, one of the things that I like best about my job is the opportunity to share what I have learned with others. Alwyn and Rachel Cosgrove have created a very special place, and they have given me more opportunities to grow and learn than I could have imagined when I first started at Results Fitness back in late 2006. They embody the idea that to be your best, you must learn from the best, and they spared no expense to make this a reality at Results Fitness. One of our core values is to constantly learn and improve, and this is what the Cosgroves are all about.

The highest compliment that I can pay them is that I know that they truly care, and this is always evident. They have invested so much money and time in me and my education that it would require pages and pages to list it all and I would quickly run out of space. Thank you for your tireless dedication and all the things you both taught me. I truly appreciate the drive to push me to become my best and I thank you both for all the opportunities you gave me and all the lessons you taught me. You made me a better person and even though you are both younger than me, I want to grow up to be like you one day.

To my teammates and clients at Results Fitness for the past 14 years. Thank you for all of your support and for putting up with me all these years. I hope you all know how deeply I care about what we do, this special little place, and the moments we all share.

To my wife, Angela, thank you for your loving support as I have pursued my passion. Through it all, we can always count on each other. You are my favorite journey over the past 25 years.

PART I

Programming:
Going Beyond the Basics

CHAPTER 1

Programmed Response

The moment Alwyn became self-actualized with regard to programming was when he realized that he could make an adaptation happen by directing the process physiologically, an approach otherwise known as, "results by design, not by coincidence." Specific and intentional results could be part of the plan, which is far different than simply doing a random training session and waiting to see what might happen. The process of imposing an appropriate stressor and expecting an adaption could be demonstrable and repeatable; this is the SAID (Specific Adaptation to Imposed Demands) principle in action. Training, in a nutshell, is simply imposing an appropriate stressor on the body, and the body adapting to it during the recovery period. The type of adaption can be selected and manipulated depending on the type of stressor imposed. This is programming with a purpose and a process.

As previously mentioned, fitness professionals are time constrained. The hourly and daily schedules of most fitness professionals a unlike that of most other professions. It is not for the faint of heart. While most of the world tends to work the typical 8 to 5, Monday through Friday, fitness professionals often work split shifts between the hours of 5 a.m. (or even earlier) to 12 p.m. and from 3 p.m. to 9 p.m. This is because we need to fill our schedules with the people who just happen to work the typical 8 to 5! This is the tradeoff for pursuing our passion of helping others and doing what we love.

Coaching clients one-on-one is how we make this happen, and unless you are creating and being paid for programming, you probably aren't earning money during the times that you are doing client programming. In addition, a coaching schedule doesn't leave a lot of time in the day for designing programs, especially, the "cooking from scratch" type.

This is not a justification for poor programming or for flying by the seat of your pants (and making stuff up as you go), but as busy professionals, time is always going to be a limiting factor and a bottleneck. This leaves you in a real quandary since good programming is so important. The question we must ask ourselves is, "How can we deal with time constraints and still deliver the goods?"

The answer is that we can do some front-end work by planning some courses in advance and then making small adjustments to these plans with additional information by "platooning" our programming based upon client goals and training age.

The mindset must be to think of the process of programming as a solution to a problem. Programming *is* simply problem solving, and it is a skill that can be taught and learned. That said, it does require experience and practice to improve. This can take precious time and since this time is a limiting factor, the next best option is to use a premade designed program. But not just any program will do! You can't just do anything and get the intended results. You need to choose wisely.

I know, I know, you're thinking that this can't be as good as a specialized and custom program designed by a master programming craftsman for a particular individual. This may or may not be true as we discussed previously. But one thing is certain: Following a plan is better than not following a plan at all. Similarly, it's better to have an idea how to get to a specific destination on a road trip, rather than taking off in any direction and hoping to end up there. At the very least, a pre-designed program will give you the desired structure and outline to get you going in the right direction.

To deliver desired results, you must follow a program that contains a logical sequence of steps with properly formatted programming variables unique to each client.

In the upcoming chapters, we share several of these preplanned programs (and discuss how to choose them) so that you can use them with your clients with very little, if any, modifications needed. That said, we also explain how to adjust as needed in chapter 3.

Our overall purpose is to introduce a process that streamlines your time and effort to consistently deliver results to your client. This requires the use of templates and preplanned programs with exercises that are already selected.

One of the major criticisms of using templates is that it is a cookie-cutter type of approach. I think that a lot of this criticism is related to how people define *templates*. In fitness and training world, we view the term template as simply an outline or a "skeleton" that can be changed and modified as needed for the client in front of you. Programmers misuse templates when they rigidly adhere to them with zero flexibility. They are figuratively not chiseled in stone, but in pencil. This means that things can be erased and changed if needed. Perhaps the problem lies with the word *template*. Be sure to understand going forward that templates are flexible, not rigid!

We like to say that you shouldn't try to fit the individual to the template, but you should fit the chosen template to the individual. In addition, you should have templates or outlines for many different goals and training ages, not just one template that you rigidly try to fit all of your clients into. Templates are the key to being time efficient.

Let's revisit the four steps of program design that we introduced in the preface:

1. Determine our goal.
2. Determine our starting point (training status).
3. Determine our time frame.
4. Plan backward and execute forward.

Now let's elaborate on these steps and delve into the process in greater detail. Our intent is to show you the principles that the upcoming programs are based on and to give further insight to the process that was used to formulate them.

"Give a man a fish and you feed him for a day. Teach a man to fish and you feed him for a lifetime." This old adage is fairly cliché but it's a fitting sentiment when it comes to learning and understanding how to program. We are not going to give you "the fish" so to speak, but we are going to explain how we fished. This is to provide empowerment with the programs provided.

Step 1: Determine Our Goal

Note that this first step states *our* goal. This wording is deliberate because the client and coach are about to embark on a journey together.

In *Alice in Wonderland*, there is an exchange between Alice and the Cheshire Cat in which the cat says to Alice (paraphrased), "If you don't know where you are going, any road can take you there" (Carroll, Haughton, and Carroll, 2009). In order to write an effective training program, we have to know a person's goal and what brought them to you. Otherwise we are only guessing and assuming. I am sure you already know what they say about assumptions…

So, what's the goal?

We have to begin with the end destination in mind. It's the first question in the program design process and it guides all of our decisions; we can't ever lose sight of it. As famed strength coach and iron philosopher Dan John says, "The goal is to keep the goal the goal."

We tend to like specific goals the best. Many productivity experts are proponents of the concept of SMART goals. This stands for Specific, Measurable, Attainable, Relevant, and Time-based. For example, a client's SMART goal may be to lose 20 pounds (9 kg) of body fat in eight months for an upcoming wedding. Let's break this down:

- This goal is *specific* because the client has indicated the amount of body fat to lose.
- It is a *measurable* and trackable amount.
- It is realistic and *attainable* in the time available.
- It is *relevant* because the emotional "why" attached to it relates to wanting to look good for a wedding. *Pro-tip*: it is always important to ask "why?" when goal-setting.
- Lastly, it is *time-based* because we have a hard deadline of eight months.

We know what direction our training is going to go in.

I know what you're thinking, "What if they have more than one goal?" Can you have more than one goal? Of course, but you can only have one priority! Using the same client as above, let's say they have the following multiple goals:

- Deadlift 300 pounds (136 kg) in 12 months
- Lose 20 pounds (9 kg) of body fat in eight months
- Complete a local triathlon in 11 months

Ask your client to prioritize the goals and then focus on one thing at time. We can eventually attain all of these goals, but we can't do them very well all at once. As our friend and colleague Eric Cressey often states, "You can't ride two horses with one butt."

Step 2: Determine Our Starting Point (Training Status)

Can you tell me how to get to Miami? I'm sure you can, but the directions you give me are going to be different if I am starting in Los Angeles or if I am starting in New York City. They will be different still if I am starting in Jacksonville. In order to formulate any training plan we first have to know the endpoint (i.e., the goal) and the starting point.

We determine our starting point by looking at several factors, the client's current state of physical preparedness, and the client's current training age and accurate training history.

Current State of Physical Preparedness

First, we need to assess the client's current state of physical preparedness, including general movement quality on a battery of basic movements. To paraphrase physical therapist Charlie Weingroff, "The main goal is to use some type of a preexercise screen to tell us if the joints can get into the positions we are asking of them to be able to absorb and adapt to stress."

Fitness expert Paul Chek has a great quote: "If you are not assessing, you are guessing." But which assessment do you use? There are quite a few movement screens and assessments that we like. In the end, it's less important which one you use, but that you use something formalized so it can be repeatable and reliable. It also needs to directly impact your programming decisions, otherwise you are just collecting data. You have to use the data or there is no real point in obtaining it. We will present a battery of physical assessments that are simple to use and that will help you determine a starting point so the client can experience success with early wins, and you can get maximum buy-in from them.

Current Training Age and Accurate Training History

Next, we qualify our client's current training age and obtain an accurate training history, which can be quite challenging to do. We do this in an unconventional way by taking something that has been traditionally very subjective, and make it as objective as possible. In chapter 2, you will see how we determine the training level of our client using a rubric to score a handful of general and specific questions.

The starting point also needs to include the typical PAR-Q (Physical Activity Readiness Questionnaire) questions to determine if the client has any possible red flag medical contraindications such as cardiac conditions, past injuries, surgeries, pain history, or medications. This information can greatly affect programming decisions, so it needs to be included when determining the starting point.

Step 3: Determine Our Time Frame

Time is a forgotten factor. We often assume the client's available time without asking. This is a big mistake.

There are three time-based questions that factor strongly into our programming decisions:

1. How long do we have to reach the stated goal?
2. How many days per week is the client available to train?
3. On these days, how many hours are available for training?

The answer to the first question will usually be included in step 1 of our programming process.

The second question must be asked and not assumed. You can write the world's greatest five-day per-week training plan, complete with recovery days and the perfect cardio sessions, but what do you do if your client only has two to three days to train each week? You're going to have to tear up your plan and start over.

The third and final question is critical as well. What if you plan for one-hour sessions but your client only has a half hour to train at each session? If we're lucky, we get an hour per session, two to three days per week with our clients, and anything more than that is gravy but not typical. This is the reality of our busy world.

One of the reasons that typical bodybuilding splits don't work for most of our clients is that the frequency of exposure to the movement patterns, and therefore the muscle groups, isn't enough to drive the adaptions that we are seeking. The old three days on, one day off program that bodybuilders use just doesn't cut the mustard for the typical client since they don't have six days per week available to invest in training.

Step 4: Plan Backward and Execute Forward

Start with the end in mind. We previously stated that the biggest mistake rookie programmers make with regards to programming is that they start with exercise selection and go forward from there. We would consider this to be a suboptimal approach; there are more important factors to consider prior to exercise choices to achieve the adaptations we are seeking.

Here are the key variables that we manipulate in our training programs (listed in order of importance):

Repetitions

Sets

Loading

Tempo

Rest Periods

Exercise Selection (most individualized)

The first three items are components of training volume or workload which is our primary training stressor. Repetitions are without a doubt, the primary variable that we manipulate in our training plans.

Keep in mind that just because exercise selection is listed last doesn't mean that it is not important, it only means that it is less important than the variables above it. When it comes to personalization of programming, we actually consider exercise selection to be the variable that offers the most individualization. In later chapters, we discuss all of these variables in much greater detail and how to apply them in our programming.

Figure 1.1 shows how our planning process is broken down.

To paraphrase noted periodization researcher Dr. Mike Zourdos of Florida Atlantic University, "All periodization is integrated." These concepts do not function completely independently of each other; they are overarching themes of a training outline and

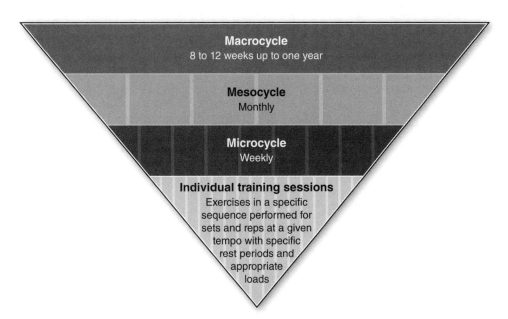

Figure 1.1 Big picture to small picture planning process.

Basic Programming Terminology

Before we get too far, let's put forward some terminology that we are going to use in our programming so that we are all on the same page.

- *The program (Macrocycle)*: The complete training plan—the outline of the sequence of monthly training blocks, which could be a year or more, or as little as two months.
- *Phase (Mesocycle)*: The four to six week training blocks consisting of a series of training weeks.
- *Training week (Microcycle)*: The sequence of training days for the week.
- *Training day/session:* Each individual workout day.

---

elements of many of these concepts are present in a big picture plan. Now let's explain these concepts with some examples to give some context behind this process.

Planning Macrocycles

When we outline our macrocycles (with respect to repetitions) we can choose from several different overarching themes, but there are the following common types:

Linear Periodization

Linear periodization involves a linear progression as we decrease reps and increase load, representing an inverse relationship between volume and intensity. Typically, the variables in this model (as laid out at the beginning of step 4) change with each mesocycle. As an example, take a look at table 1.1.

Table 1.1 Linear Periodization

Phase	Weeks	Repetitions
Phase 1	Weeks 1-3	12 reps
Phase 2	Weeks 4-6	10 reps
Phase 3	Weeks 7-9	8 reps
Phase 4	Weeks 10-12	6 reps

Nonlinear Alternating Periodization

Nonlinear alternating periodization involves alternating between volume and intensity phases. As an example, take a look at table 1.2.

Table 1.2 Nonlinear Alternating Periodization

Phase	Weeks	Repetitions
Phase 1	Weeks 1-4	15 reps (volume)
Phase 2	Weeks 5-8	10 reps (intensity)
Phase 3	Weeks 9-12	12 reps (volume)
Phase 4	Weeks 13-16	8 reps (intensity)

Daily Undulating Periodization

Daily undulating periodization (DUP) involves alternating between volume and intensity on a session-by-session basis within the same training week (or on a weekly basis). Again, repetitions and therefore intensity are periodized which in turn, affects volume. There are many permutations of this. As an example, take a look at table 1.3 where training takes place three days per week on Monday, Wednesday, and Friday.

Table 1.3 Daily Undulating Periodization

Phase	Weeks	Repetitions
Phase 1	Weeks 1-4	M: 15 reps, W: 12 reps, F: 10 reps
Phase 2	Weeks 5-8	M: 12 reps, W: 10 reps, F: 8 reps
Phase 3	Weeks 9-12	M: 10 reps, W: 8 reps, F: 6 reps

Planning Mesocycles/Phases

When we plan our mesocycles, we need to lay out what each training phase sequence (basically the month of training) will specifically look like. Table 1.4 provides a breakdown of Phase 1 of our linear periodization plan from above and what it could potentially look like when laid out for an entire month if the client is training three times per week on an A and B session full-body split.

Table 1.4 Linear Periodization: Sample Mesocycle Outline for Phase 1

Week	Monday	Wednesday	Friday
Week 1	Day A: 12 reps	Day B: 12 reps	Day A: 12 reps
Week 2	Day B: 12 reps	Day A: 12 reps	Day B: 12 reps
Week 3	Day A: 12 reps	Day B: 12 reps	Day A: 12 reps
Week 4	Day B: 12 reps	Day A: 12 reps	Day B: 12 reps

Table 1.5 provides an outline for a DUP plan mesocycle, and breaks down the rep sequencing in each session for each of the four weeks of the sample mesocycle.

Table 1.5 Daily Undulating Periodization: Sample Mesocycle Outline

Week	Monday	Wednesday	Friday
Week 1	Day A: 5 reps	Day B: 15 reps	Day A: 10 reps
Week 2	Day B: 5 reps	Day A: 15 reps	Day B: 10 reps
Week 3	Day A: 5 reps	Day B: 15 reps	Day A: 10 reps
Week 4	Day B: 5 reps	Day A: 15 reps	Day B: 10 reps

Planning Microcycles and Training Weeks/Sessions

As we further subdivide our plan, we take each session of the week and outline it in greater detail to the microlevel. To start, note that all the resistance training sessions are composed of the following component parts (each component will be described in detail in the next chapter):

RAMP (range of motion, activation, movement preparation)
Core
Power and elasticity or combination and rotation
Strength and resistance training
Energy system training
Regeneration

Most of our clients have an hour to train so we place time caps on each of these components. The breakdown of an hour typically looks like the following:

RAMP: 0:00 to 0:15
Core: 0:15 to 0:22
Power and elasticity or combination and rotation: 0:22 to 0:27
Strength and resistance: 0:27 to 0:57
Energy system: 0:57 to 1:00+ (if time allows)

We then break down each constituent part of these components and lay out the details of each session. Table 1.6 shows what a day A and day B program may look like when broken down into the movement patterns for the resistance training component. From here we plan the reps, sets, tempos, and rest periods, for this microcycle, and finish with specific exercises. Now we have a plan!

Table 1.6 Strength Training Movement Pattern Allocation: Sample Microcycle

Day A: full body	Day B: full body
1A Squat pattern (symmetrical stance) 1B Pull pattern	1A Hinge pattern (symmetrical stance) 1B Push pattern
2A Hinge pattern (asymmetrical or single-leg stance) 2B Push pattern	2A Squat pattern (asymmetrical or single-leg stance) 2B Pull pattern

There you have it: A step-by-step and systematic approach to program design. The main purpose of this chapter was to emphasize the most important concept that we want you take away from this book, the concept of planning. Remember, we begin with the big picture in mind and then break things down to the individual workout or training session level. What we don't do is start with the mentality of "What exercises am I going to do with this person?"

CHAPTER 2

Accurately Assessing Current Training Status

As we learned in the previous chapter, step 1 in our four-step program design process is to determine the client goals. Once these have been set, the next step is to establish our starting point. An assessment is simply a method of establishing where the client is, with respect to where they want to go, and it answers the question of where to start when it comes to program design. You begin with an assessment to establish a hierarchy of client needs and look for any red flags (e.g., injuries) or other limiting factors that could prevent progress.

At our facility, when a potential new client comes in for the first time, we perform what we call a *strategy session*. This allows us to go through our investigative process to determine their individual starting point. The session lasts about an hour and consists of the following four steps:

1. Sitting down to determine training goals.

2. Asking specific and thorough questions about health and medical history, documenting all the information. This would include specifics about dates and types of surgeries, past injuries, heart conditions, current medications, and any other chronic conditions that are relevant to training.

3. Asking specific interview questions about previous training history and preferences. This is where we use our rubric to qualify training age.

4. Conducting the Functional Movement Screen (FMS) to assess a fundamental movement pattern baseline.

In this chapter we investigate two primary areas to determine this starting point: a qualification of the client's current training age, and an assessment of the client's current state of physical preparedness and fundamental movement quality. We discuss how to use the information from the assessments and apply it to programming.

Qualifying Training Age

One of the more challenging things to do in the programming process is to accurately determine a client's training age and where they fall on the training age continuum (see figure 2.1). This is a source of much debate and opinion. It's not very challenging to classify or rank a beginner that is at the very start of this continuum. If someone has no experience in resistance training, you know that the person in front of you is

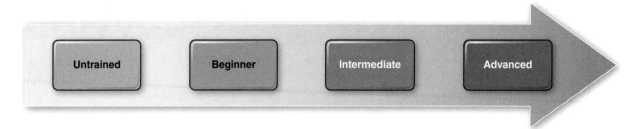

Figure 2.1   Training age continuum.

a beginner because they are untrained, but beyond that, it's often much less cut and dried. This is because there is much more involved than simply asking the question, "How long have you been resistance training?"

What if a client has two or more years of resistance training experience? Are they now categorized as advanced or are they only an intermediate? Could the client still be a beginner? That answer of *two years* must be qualified and given context.

In our opinion, training age isn't simply about the total amount of time that you have been training, it's more about the time that you have spent performing *quality* training. The "quantity of quality" is what matters when determining training age. We are going to explain how we apply this context and qualify this status at our facility. It's certainly not the only way, but it does provide some clarity to the process.

We can ascertain a solid estimation of training age, but we are never going be exact because there is always some degree of subjectivity. We work to minimize the degree of subjectivity by providing tools and knowledge to guide us on where to begin with a client when it comes to the programming options provided later on in the book.

Our programming options funnel our clients into one of two groups:

- Beginner to Intermediate
- Advanced

Just about everyone beyond the true beginner likes to fancy themselves as being advanced, or, at the very least, being an intermediate. The problem is that no one wants to be labeled a beginner. In reality, most people that believe they are advanced are far less advanced than they think they are. Our ego often gets in the way because there is a negative stigma associated with the idea of being a beginner and needing to focus on the basics. People often feel that this is too remedial. This mistake can come back to haunt you if you dive into training options that are unnecessary or that you are underprepared for, which can end up impeding your progress.

But guess what? Being a beginner is actually a great thing, so it's wise to embrace it rather than fight it. It's a chance to master the basics. The best in the world are often the best because they perform the basics better than others. Being a beginner means that you have the potential to make a great amount of progress in a reasonably short amount of time because your ceiling for adaptation is higher than that of the advanced person. This simply means that if you haven't had many adaptations to proper resistance training, you have a lot of room to improve. This should get a person very excited. The gains that occur during this time can be incredible, and it builds a lot of buy in from clients due to the rapid progress that they can make.

"If something's new to you, you're a beginner," Mark Verstegen, the founder of EXOS, has said. Mark's quote is an elegant truth and it also helps to soothe the ego problem because it takes the ego out of it. It's also the simplest filter that trumps everything else (even our rubric later in this chapter). We all have things that are new to us and when we accept this, we realize that it's safe and it's okay to be a beginner. Another training and coaching reality is that most of the clients that come to see us are going to be beginners. Very few clients that seek to work with a trainer will start out as advanced trainees.

But let's say that you do have a client who has been training as a recreational competitive powerlifter for more than 15 years and decides to take some time away from powerlifting to really concentrate on fat-loss programming. Guess what? No matter how advanced the powerlifter may be, we would still assign this client to a beginner fat-loss program. Why? Because even someone very strong is underprepared to jump into an advanced fat-loss program; a person needs to build up to it progressively. It's new, and being a beginner in fat-loss training methods, the client doesn't need unnecessary programming complexity. There will be more return on training investment using simpler means.

Figure 2.2 shows a scoring rubric that we have created to help us objectively qualify a client's training age as it pertains primarily to resistance training. A rubric is simply a descriptive scoring scheme. We have listed qualifying statements for each potential score, but you must use your best judgement when selecting the score. We assign a value to each of the six questions using a score of 1, 2, or 3, and then calculate the scores to the answers of each of the six questions. We use this total to assign the client to the beginner to intermediate category or to the advanced category to determine the proper training program starting point.

Figure 2.2   Training Age Scoring Rubric

Question 1: What is the client's resistance training experience?	Score
a. This will be the client's first experience with a structured and supervised resistance training program, *or* the client has resistance training experience but has never followed a structured program and has never worked with a coach on a sensible[1] training program.	1 point
b. The client has previously trained consistently for a period of 6 mo-2 years following a sensible training and structured program working with a qualified coach.	2 points
c. The client has been training seriously and following sensible training programming for a period of more than 2 years.	3 points
Question 2: At this current point in time, when was the last time the client resistance trained consistently?[2]	
a. This is the client's first experience with resistance training, *or* it has been more than 3 mo since last training.	1 point
b. The client was consistently resistance training 1-2 wk ago.	2 points
c. The client is regularly resistance training 2-4 times per wk at this current point in time.	3 points
Question 3: What is the client's current general daily activity level?[3]	
a. The client is completely sedentary (e.g., desk job or very little overall daily activity).	1 point
b. The client is somewhat active (e.g., weekend warrior–type recreational athlete or regular long hikes on weekend).	2 points
c. The client is very active (almost daily physical exercise or sport of some sort, or a physically active job).	3 points
Question 4: What is the client's athletic background or competitive sports background?[4]	
a. The client has no athletic background or participated in one sport growing up and in high school.	1 point
b. The client played more than one sport in high school.	2 points
c. The client participated in college athletics or played multiple sports through high school or beyond.	3 points

(continued)

Figure 2.2 Training Age Scoring Rubric *(continued)*

Question 5: What is the client's current strength level?[5]	
a. The client is unable to perform a properly executed squat or a deadlift with a load equivalent to body-weight (or has never performed the movements), or cannot perform a bodyweight chin-up or multiple push-ups with proper technique (or has never performed the movements).	1 point
b. The client is capable of a properly executed squat or a deadlift with a load equivalent to bodyweight, or capable of multiple repetitions of bodyweight chin-ups and push-ups.	2 points
c. The client is capable of a properly executed squat or a deadlift with a load equivalent to 1.5 times bodyweight or greater, can perform externally loaded chin-ups, can bench press with a load equivalent to bodyweight, or can perform overhead press with a load that is .75 times bodyweight.	3 points
Question 6: What is the client's Functional Movement Screen (FMS) baseline score?[6]	
a. FMS total score is lower than 13 with one or more asymmetries (in one of the tests).	1 point
b. FMS total score of 14-16 with no asymmetries.	2 points
c. FMS total score of 17 or above with no asymmetries.	3 points

Notes:

[1]In this context, *sensible training* means that the client has trained in a manner that is in line with of two of our key principles: (1) Training has focused on training movements, not muscles (utilizing most if not all of the primal movements that we will discuss in chapter 3), and (2) they have used multijoint compound movements in their training as priority (i.e., not machine-based), adhering to proper standards of performance.

[2]Even if someone has some degree of sensible training under their belt, but they haven't trained for the past three months, assign that person a score of 1 because they are currently in a detrained state.

[3]This question gives us a sense of how much activity someone is presently doing and suggests their general state of pre-paredness for physical activity. It helps to determine how to dose the training early on, because someone who is completely sedentary will be likely to incur more muscle damage and soreness compared to someone who has a physically active job or performs daily exercise.

[4]This question gives us a sense of the size of the movement motor learning "pool" that someone has to draw from. Generally, we have observed that the more diverse a sports backgrounds, the easier time the client will have learning new motor skills.

[5]Should you formally test a client's strength level prior to implementing a training plan? You certainly can if someone is pre-pared for it. We feel that you can make pretty good estimations of strength based on the answers to the previous questions on the rubric without having to directly test it prior to training (there are always some exceptions). The purpose of question 5 isn't to assign strength achievement standards, but to give clarity to the proper training level by whether or not the client scored a 1 or a 3 on this qualifier.

[6]You will not be able to actually answer this question until step 4 of the strategy session is completed. We don't use the FMS to test how much someone can do, we use it to rate and rank the quality of the movement. It gives us a part of the picture, but not the whole picture. Alwyn has previously stated in a seminar: "Just because you move well doesn't mean that you need an advanced program." Someone who scores really high on the screen moves well and has great mobility and stability. Training age and experience with any given exercise must always be considered first when prescribing any exercise, and if the client *does not* move well, entry level exercises and programming should be used to begin.

Once we have finished the strategy session, we calculate the scores of our training age assessment and place the client into the appropriate training level category based on their score (see table 2.1). A score of less than 15 would place the client in the beginner to intermediate category. A score of 15 or above could place them in the advanced group, starting with the advanced programming options if desired, but it would not be wrong to go with the beginner to intermediate option; the client would more than likely benefit from this choice. Also, don't let the client make the mistake of confusing a beginner program that looks fairly simple with being easy. A beginner program can be very challenging given the properly assigned loads and exercises; the loads (i.e., intensities assigned) and exercises will be the highly individualized portion of the programming.

Table 2.1 Training Age Scoring

Total score	Potential training age
6-10 total points =	Beginner training age
11-14 total points =	Intermediate training age
15-18 total points =	Advanced training age

Evaluating Movement Quality

The fourth and final step of our strategy session is the movement portion. For this, we have found Gray Cook and Lee Burton's Functional Movement Screen (2010) to be the most effective method of evaluating fundamental movement quality. It consists of seven different screening tests that cover the entire body. Our facility was one of the first implementers of the screen in the private sector, and we have been using it for over 15 years. Frankly, we have never found anything that works better to give us the information we need. It allows us to have an assessment system that our entire staff can follow to design an effective program. We have tried to use more complex forms of assessment but later realized that a screen of the basic functional movements tells us almost everything we need to know for programming as a fitness coach.

Pros of a Formalized Movement Assessment

There has recently been a considerable amount of debate regarding movement assessment in the fitness industry. Some coaches are for it, some are against it. The truth is that just about all fitness professionals assess whether they realize it or not. The main difference is whether one uses a formal or informal assessment at the intake of a new client.

We feel that a formalized movement assessment is critical as part of our system. We need to have the ability to replicate the assessment process so we can easily teach it to other coaches as part of our programming model. This allows multiple coaches to have the ability to perform the assessment, we get consistent and reliable findings, and we all speak the same language.

Standardized movement assessment is not supposed to replace the skilled eye of an experienced coach or clinician. It aims to provide measurement and objectivity to some elements of performance and human movement. We prefer to use all the essential tools at our disposal instead of only some of them. Whether you buy into formal assessments or informal assessments, once again in the words of Paul Chek, "If you are not assessing, you're guessing."

Our program is only as good as the assessment. A doctor wouldn't prescribe a drug or perform a surgery until you have been diagnosed. In our opinion, a fitness program is not too different. An ongoing joke with our staff is that we cannot write a poor program. We can only write a good program that is based on a poor assessment. If the assessment is incorrect, then every training-based decision is based on an incorrect starting point.

Before we go too much further, we should probably differentiate between the *screen* and *assessment* because these terms can be somewhat confusing at times. At a seminar several years ago, FMS cofounder Lee Burton was presenting about the FMS and stated that the difference between the two terms is that "a screen simply tells you that

---

Stay in Your Lane and Know Your Own Limitations

A question often arises as to when a performance coach is overstepping a boundary and crossing the line into the realm of a medical clinician. If we are to draw a line, it should be drawn at the presentation of serious pain. The first principle of training is to "do no harm." Refer a client that presents with pain to a qualified medical professional. Fitness professionals are not typically trained to treat pain and are more than likely crossing a line when they attempt to do so. Do these lines get blurred on occasion? Most certainly, but always use your best judgment to know when to refer out. *If there is any doubt, refer out.* Fitness professionals should be trained and should be knowledgeable enough to correct muscular imbalances, faulty movement patterns, and, most importantly, address the client's goals with respect to these things. A coach must be mindful of his or her own limitations and be completely aware of overstepping boundaries. We feel that Boston-based coach Tony Bonvechio sums it up really well when he states, "It's our job as coaches to teach and coach good movement, not to treat pain."

---

something is wrong, and an assessment tells you *what* is wrong." He likens screening to taking blood pressure. If someone has high blood pressure, you know that something is wrong, but you don't know what specifically is wrong without further investigation. Screening is the first step. Going forward we use the terms interchangeably, but please realize that there can be a distinction. The other reason that we use the word assessment is that the word *screening* doesn't rhyme as well with *guessing*.

Introduction to the Functional Movement Screen

Many of you may be quite familiar with Gray Cook and Lee Burton's Functional Movement Screen (2010). Over the past 15 years that we have used the FMS, it has been awesome to see its growth and wide acceptance. For the uninitiated, the following is an explanation and brief history of the movement screen from the FMS level one manual:

"The Functional Movement Screen captures fundamental movements, motor control within movement patterns, and competence of basic movements uncomplicated by specific skills. It will determine the greatest areas of movement deficiency, demonstrate limitations or asymmetries, and eventually correlate these with an outcome. Once you find the greatest asymmetry or deficiency, you can use additional screens that are more precise if needed.

The original idea of the screen was to portray movement-pattern quality with a simple grading system of movement appraisal; it's not intended to diagnose or measure isolated joint movement. Attempting to measure in isolation does a disservice to the pattern—the body is too complex to take isolated movements seriously in the initial stages of screening.

This system was developed to rate and rank movement patterns in high school athletes, in an effort to determine who was ready to engage in higher-level activities in the weight room and on the field. However, during the two-year refining process, we discovered uses well beyond the original intended purpose, the information gathered from its use has broadened our scope of corrective exercise, training and rehabilitation. The screen has taught us how to use it, and helped us gain timely and valuable feedback from our attempts at movement correction.

Our collective expertise has come from working against the screen's standard, not from modifying the screen every time things got confusing or inconvenient. We have changed the way we look at the screen data many times, but we have not changed the way we collect the information. In a way, this work represents our evolution, not that of the screen. The screen patiently waited for us to see and understand all it was providing in return for about 10 minutes worth of time.

The FMS is comprised of seven movement tests that require a balance of mobility and stability. The patterns used provide observable performance of basic mobility and stability movements by placing clients in positions where weaknesses, imbalances, asymmetries and limitations become noticeable by a trained health and fitness professional.

When the screen's movements mimic athletic moves, it is merely coincidence. The screen is not a training tool, nor is it a competition tool. It's purely an instrument for rating and ranking movements.

The screen's usefulness is its simplicity, practicality and ability to fill a void in the toolbox we use to judge performance and durability. It is not intended to determine why a dysfunctional or faulty movement pattern exists. Instead, it's a discovery of which patterns are problematic. The FMS exposes dysfunction or pain—or both— within basic movement patterns.

Many people are able to perform a wide range of activities, yet are unable to efficiently execute the movements in the screen. Those who score poorly on the screens are using compensatory movement patterns during regular activities. If these compensations continue, suboptimal movement patterns are reinforced, leading to poor biomechanics and possibly contributing to a future injury.

The public's knowledge of the intricacies of the FMS is minimal at best. To introduce your client to the process, suggest a visit to the Functional Movement Systems website at FunctionalMovement.com."[1]

The Functional Movement Screen Tests

According to Richard Schmidt in his book *Motor Learning and Performance* (1991), the body can only do certain things: squat, lunge, bend, push, pull, twist and gait. The Functional Movement Screen demonstrates the client's ability to perform a generic and primal version of these movements, which is why we find it to be so valuable. The FMS consists of the following seven formalized tests:

1. Deep squat (DS)
2. Hurdle step (HS)
3. Inline lunge (ILL)
4. Shoulder mobility (SM)
5. Active straight leg raise (ASLR)
6. Trunk stability push-up (TSPU)
7. Rotational stability (RS)

Each of these is scored on a scale of 0 to 3 based on the quality of the movement (a 0 being reserved for a finding of painful movement). There can only be one of four possible findings on each of the seven tests:

---

[1]Reprinted with permission of Functional Movement Systems.

3—Optimal

2—Acceptable

1—Dysfunctional

0—Painful

A perfect total score on the screen is a 21 (receiving a 3 on all seven tests), but don't misunderstand that the goal is for everyone to get a 21. Instead, a score of 14 with no gross asymmetries is the goal, because it means that the client has good, clean movement and minimized risk factors. Calculating asymmetries can be confusing in tests that compare both sides of the body. The FMS recognizes some degree of natural asymmetry within the scoring criteria. It attempts to point out gross or excessive asymmetries as being a potential warning sign. Brett Jones, a staff member for the Functional Movement Systems, has stated that,

"some trainers get stuck in the 'corrective whirlpool' where they are always trying to correct something and are holding back from progressing into conditioning. All 2s, no asymmetries, appears to be a very good level (based on the research with military and NFL), and while we can always continue with some movement prep and work on a pattern—if you are all 2s, without asymmetry, then your client should be progressing. The goal is not to be a 21."[2]

For specifics on how to score the FMS and descriptions of how to perform each individual test, readers are directed to the book *Movement* by Gray Cook and colleagues (2010) or www.functionalmovement.com. An in-depth exploration of the FMS is not only an entirely different book (that's why we defer to Cook) but is also typically a two- or three-day workshop to learn how to apply the screen, score in practice, and apply specific corrective exercises for each of the tests.

Here we apply values to the client's movement patterns:

- *3*—The client can cleanly execute the pattern. The coach trains the pattern.
- *2*—The client can execute the pattern with some degree of compensation. The coach trains the pattern but may need to continue to work with the client to improve the pattern.
- *1*—The client cannot cleanly execute the pattern; the pattern is significantly limited or dysfunctional. The coach corrects the pattern—does not externally load that particular pattern and does not train it in aggressive fashion. Instead, the coach initially focuses on "patterning the movement" to get it up to snuff.
- *0*—Pain is evident in the client. The coach refers the client to a qualified medical professional for diagnosis, evaluation, or rehab as warranted.

As mentioned we are mainly concerned with the scores of 0, 1, and 2. From a programming standpoint, there is not much distinction between the score of 2 and 3 because a score of 2 indicates that the client is cleared to train the pattern in question. The FMS is not a performance test—it's a movement quality test that establishes a client's bodyweight competency. It indicates competency at a given movement, not how much or how many times a movement can be performed.

FMS Scores and General Exercise Programming Indications

Table 2.2 provides general procedures for how we go about applying the results of the FMS to our programming model in our resistance and core training components. Keep in mind that the following is not intended to be exhaustive for all scenarios but are primarily intended to provide guidelines and show rationale.

[2]Used with permission of Brett Jones.

Table 2.2   Functional Movement Screen

	FMS TEST: DEEP SQUAT (DS)	
	APPLIED TO SQUAT SUBCATEGORY: SYMMETRICAL (PARALLEL) STANCE	
	FMS score	**General indications and procedures based on score**
	1	Address mobility and stability needs and potentially start this progression with an assisted squat or a bodyweight box squat. Focus on patterning proper movement. Avoid externally loaded squat patterns if score is a 1.
	2	Train the movement starting with the goblet squat or regress a level depending on client training age and proficiency.
	3	Train the movement starting with the goblet squat or a more advanced level exercise progression depending on training age and strength levels.
	0	Avoid this pattern and refer client to medical professional for a diagnosis as warranted. Substitute the pattern with a nonpainful pattern.
	FMS TEST: INLINE LUNGE (ILL)	
	APPLIED TO SQUAT SUBCATEGORY: ASYMMETRICAL (SPLIT) STANCE	
	FMS score	**General indications and procedures based on score**
	1	Address mobility and stability needs and potentially start with an assisted bottoms-up split squat. Avoid externally loaded split squat exercises in this category if score is a 1. Focus on utilizing half-kneeling exercise postures in training with the other movement patterns as well.
	2	Train the movement starting with the goblet split squat or regress a level depending on client training age and proficiency.
	3	Train the movement starting with the goblet split squat or a more advanced level exercise progression depending on training age and strength levels.
	0	Avoid this pattern and refer client to medical professional for a diagnosis as warranted. Substitute the pattern with a nonpainful pattern.
	FMS TEST: HURDLE STEP (HS)	
	APPLIED TO SQUAT AND HIP HINGE SUBCATEGORY: SINGLE-LEG STANCE	
	FMS score	**General indications and procedures based on score**
	1	Address mobility and stability needs and start with low bodyweight step-up in the squat subcategory of single-leg stance, and assisted or bodyweight single-leg Romanian deadlift in the hinge subcategory of single-leg stance. Avoid externally loaded single-leg stance exercises in these exercise subcategories.
	2	Train the movement starting with goblet step-up in the squat subcategory of single-leg stance, and one-dumbbell staggered-stance Romanian deadlift in the hinge subcategory of single-leg stance or regress a level depending on client training age and proficiency.
	3	Train the movement starting with goblet step-ups in the squat subcategory of single-leg stance, and one-dumbbell staggered-stance Romanian deadlift in the hinge subcategory of single-leg stance or a more advanced level exercise progression depending on training age.
	0	Avoid this pattern and refer client to medical professional for a diagnosis as warranted. Substitute the pattern with a nonpainful pattern.

(continued)

Table 2.2 Functional Movement Screen *(continued)*

FMS TEST: SHOULDER MOBILITY (SM)		
APPLIED TO PUSH AND PULL SUBCATEGORY: VERTICAL (OVERHEAD)		
	FMS score	**General programming indications and procedures based on score**
	1	Address mobility and stability needs and potentially start with a landmine half-kneeling press or substitute another horizontal-push exercise in place of a vertical-push exercise progression. Externally loaded exercises with arms overhead should be temporarily avoided. In particular, avoid full-overhead pushing and pulling exercises where both hands are locked into position and unable to work independently of each other, such as barbell bench press or pull-up, until pattern is improved to a score of 2.
	2	Train the movement pattern subcategories starting with the appropriate exercise progression level based upon training age and proficiency.
	3	Train the movement pattern subcategories starting with the appropriate exercise progression level based upon training age and proficiency.
	0	Avoid this pattern and refer client to medical professional for a diagnosis as warranted. Substitute the category with a nonpainful pattern.

FMS TEST: ACTIVE STRAIGHT LEG RAISE (ASLR)		
APPLIED TO HIP-HINGE SUBCATEGORIES: SYMMETRICAL- (PARALLEL STANCE) AND SINGLE-LEG STANCE		
	FMS score	**General programming indications and procedures based on score**
	1	Address mobility and stability needs and start with bodyweight exercises to pattern the movement. Use the prisoner bodyweight Romanian deadlift in the hip-hinge subcategory of symmetrical stance, and the bodyweight or assisted single-leg Romanian deadlift in the hip-hinge subcategory of single-leg stance. Avoid externally loaded hip-hinge exercises in these categories.
	2	Train the movement starting with kettlebell deadlift for the hip-hinge subcategory of symmetrical stance and the one-dumbbell staggered-stance Romanian deadlift or one-dumbbell block single-leg deadlift in the hip-hinge subcategory of single-leg stance or a level down depending on client training age and proficiency.
	3	Train the movements starting with kettlebell deadlift for the hip-hinge sub-category of symmetrical stance and the one-dumbbell staggered-stance Romanian deadlift or one-dumbbell block single-leg deadlift in the hip-hinge subcategory of single-leg stance or potentially use a more advanced level exercise progression depending on training age and strength levels.
	0	Avoid this pattern and refer client to medical professional for a diagnosis as warranted. Substitute the pattern with a nonpainful pattern.

FMS TEST: TRUNK STABILITY PUSH-UP (TSPU)		
APPLIED TO CORE AND PUSH SUBCATEGORIES: ANTIEXTENSION AND PUSH HORIZONTAL AND VERTICAL		
	FMS score	**General programming indications and procedures based on score**
	1	Address stability and mobility needs and potentially start the push subcategory horizontal with an incline push-up or band-assisted push-up specifically. Core training subcategory antiextension should begin with front plank at the appropriate intensity level. High-threshold activities such as back squat and loaded overhead press are going to be potentially challenging due to the core's inability to brace well as found with a score of 1.
	2	Train the movement pattern subcategories starting with the appropriate exercise progression level based upon training age and proficiency.
	3	Train the movement pattern subcategories starting with the appropriate exercise progression level based upon training age and proficiency.
	0	Avoid this pattern and refer client to medical professional for a diagnosis as warranted. Substitute the category with a nonpainful pattern.

FMS TEST: ROTATIONAL STABILITY (RS)		
PRIMARILY APPLIED TO CORE SUBCATEGORY: ANTIROTATION		
	FMS score	**General programming indications and procedures based on score**
	1	Address stability and mobility needs and potentially start with quadruped birddog isometric hold and cable kneeling and half-kneeling antirotation press. Avoid most asymmetrical or unevenly loaded exercises that externally load only one side of the body until score is improved to a 2.
	2	Train the core antirotation subcategory starting with the appropriate exercise progression level based upon training age and proficiency.
	3	Train the core antirotation subcategory starting with the appropriate exercise progression level based upon training age and proficiency.
	0	Avoid this pattern and refer client to medical professional for a diagnosis as warranted. Substitute the category with a nonpainful pattern.

Photos courtesy of Functional Movement Systems.

The FMS and Programming Decisions

As you have seen in this chapter, the FMS mainly assists by letting us know what *not* to do rather than telling us exactly what to do. To decide what to do, we rely primarily on our exercise progressions within each category.

This may be surprising, but we don't use the FMS as the basis for writing our fitness programs. The client's goal is the primary basis for writing the program. We outline a training plan based on a client goal and with a training age in mind. We primarily use information from the FMS as a tool to determine what adjustments we need to make to our plan. The FMS helps us to make our fitness programs better by helping to fine tune them.

For instance, when we discover a 1 on any of the tests, we examine our training plan to determine the training changes we need to make in terms of exercise selection. We don't want to get paralyzed by this additional information. It's meant to help us, not freeze us in our tracks. That's why we design and lay out the plan first (based on training age) and then look at the FMS scores to see what adjustments need to be made.

Our goal is to train the whole body, but you must ask yourself the following questions:

- Does the screen suggest I eliminate something from the client's program?
- Does the screen suggest a regressed version of this movement is in order?
- Does the screen suggest that this movement is cleared for training and overload?

For example, if you are planning to assign any of the following exercises, the client needs to have met the FMS prerequisite. Just like in school where the prerequisite must be met before enrolling in a desired class: Algebra 1 needs to be taken before Algebra 2. Exercise should have established prerequisites as well (see table 2.3).

Table 2.3   Examples of FMS Exercise General Prerequisites

Exercise	Prerequisite
Loaded deadlift	ASLR = 2R/2L
Loaded squat	DS = 2
Loaded lunge	ILL = 2R/2L
Loaded overhead press	SM = 2R/2L

We have laid out our four-step process for determining a client's starting point. As part of that process, we recommend the Functional Movement Screen and we have explained how we use it to make better and more informed programming decisions. It's up to you whether or not you personally choose to use the FMS or another movement system to help you determine your client's starting point. Just make sure you use something rather than nothing at all. These are relatively simple concepts, yet very profound in application, and will save you time when programming and, most importantly, will help your clients achieve their goals.

CHAPTER 3

Progressing and Regressing Exercises on the Fly

In the words of Gray Cook, "Exercises selected should be appropriately challenging, but not too difficult." This quote has always resonated with us. We stated earlier that exercise selection is the least important exercise variable of those listed in chapter 1, but let us be very clear, this does not mean that it is not important! Exercise selection is incredibly significant, just not quite as crucial as the other programming variables.

Without a doubt, appropriate exercise selection is a learned skill. A key piece in developing this skill is having a grasp of the principles behind exercise progressions and regressions, which can often separate a great coach or programmer from a good one. Whether you use a predesigned program with preselected exercises or more of a skeleton template that has only the movement patterns listed, you need to ensure that the chosen exercise is a proper fit for the person in front of you. You must also ensure that your client is prepared for the exercise you have selected. Exercise selection is what we consider to be the most individualized aspect of programming, because we are all built a bit differently and bring our own past experiences to training, as discussed in chapter 2.

What's in a Name?

Before we get too far into the weeds of the specific aspects of exercise progressions, we must first talk about exercise nomenclature. The manner in which the exercises are named requires a bit of context because there is another system in place that we want you to be aware of.

We often joke that exercise nomenclature is the bane of our existence. Since we work together as a team, we try to execute a system that effectively communicates the name of an exercise to clients and to our coaches.

Nonstandardized exercise nomenclature is certainly a problem within the fitness industry (and in most industries, for that matter), but it may be unrealistic to expect everyone in the industry to use standardized exercise names. After all, depending on the geographical region in the United States, soda pop is referred to as *cola*, *pop*, *coke*, and *soda*!

We do believe that it is vitally important to speak the same common language within our own gym. Just like our soda pop example, it seems that almost every exercise has 5 to 10 different names within the fitness industry, but it should *not* have 5 to 10 different names within your own gym if you want to execute an effective programming and coaching system. This naming problem causes a lot of inefficiency and frustration among coaches, programmers, and clients. In our home facilities, we must ensure that we call apples *apples* if that is what we are referring to. This means that amongst your team, each exercise must have only *one* name, and everyone should consistently stick to that name.

With respect to their namesakes, we do our best to avoid naming exercises after countries or people because these names are not very descriptive to the uninitiated. That stated, and as a friendly disclaimer, we do make a few concessions with some generally known exercises, because the common name is well known by most of the industry, and in most cases we weren't able to come up with a better name. An example of this would be the Romanian deadlift (RDL).

We have also standardized how we arrange and write exercise names based on a system that our colleague Steve Di Tomaso from Envision Fitness shared with us. He uses a *position-implement-exercise* configuration when he records an exercise, and we have modified this system for our gym to *implement-position-exercise*. An example is shown in figure 3.1.

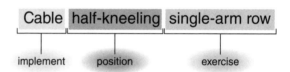

Figure 3.1 Example of implement-position-exercise naming format.

Nine Principles of Designing Exercise Progressions and Regressions

When we design exercise progressions, we place exercises into the appropriate "family trees" within various parent categories to classify the training movements with a logically developed plan to get to an end goal exercise.

Almost all exercises can be progressed or regressed depending on client ability. Without a doubt, the most common way to design exercise progressions and regressions is based on adding or reducing external load. However, it is worth mentioning that the first form of regression that we often use in practice is to simply reduce load because loads that are too heavy can be a primary problem that make an exercise too challenging. A simple load progression can occur from microcycle to microcycle without altering the exercise, or the load progression can transform the exercise to become slightly different from mesocycle to mesocycle (phase to phase) because of a new type of loading position. We provide examples of true exercise progressions later in this chapter and in our programs that follow later on in the book.

Principles of exercise regressions and progressions exist on a degree of difficulty continuum which consists of easier to harder, or less challenging to more challenging. Certain principles of load and range of motion are easier to conceptualize if one thinks in terms of easier versus harder, and other principles of stability are easier to think of in terms less challenging versus more challenging.

Table 3.1 provides a breakdown of the nine most common principles used to progress or regress exercises in terms of this continuum.

Table 3.1 Degree of Difficulty Continuum

EASIER ⟵		⟶ HARDER
Regression	**Primary progression principle**	**Progression**
Lighter	1. Load	Heavier
Wider base	2. Base of support width	Narrower base
More points of contact	3. Base of support points of contact	Fewer points of contact
More stable	4. External stability	More unstable
Closer to base of support (BOS); closer to axis of rotation (AOR)	5. Center of mass positioning (relative to base of support or axis of rotation)	Further from base of support (BOS); further from axis of rotation (AOR)
Lesser range of motion (ROM)	6. Range of motion	Greater range of motion (ROM)
Slower	7. Speed	Faster
Static	8. Movement complexity	Dynamic
Sagittal	9. Planes of motion	Frontal and transverse

Using these nine primary principles allows us to create individually challenging exercise progressions and regressions by various means. Only the first principle involves increasing or decreasing external load, so there are many other possible ways to make an exercise more or less challenging. Many of the principles use stability to vary their progressions or regressions. This simply involves the client going from a more stable to a less stable position, or vice versa, and the stability can be applied by several different means.

Many of these principles are very interconnected so some of the progressions or regressions use many of the principles and not just one. The key is that we use a logical rationale when deciding to make an exercise harder or easier.

Let's look at each of these nine principles in detail. Our examples illustrate how we apply these principles to the specific movement patterns within our training session components and exercise categories.

Load

This principle is very straightforward; we simply add load to increase the difficulty. For example, if you are doing five reps of a barbell overhead press one week with 185 pounds (84 kg), the next week you increase to 190 pounds (86 kg) with the same number of reps. Obviously, this works in the reverse manner as well to regress the exercise—reduce load to decrease the difficulty. It is worth mentioning that we can also increase or decrease the load effect of gravity by manipulating our body position or angle. An example is to perform a push-up with the hands elevated to make it easier because the angled body position puts less load on the upper body.

Base of Support Width

You can go from a wide base of support to a narrower base of support, as in a basic front plank. With your feet wide—outside shoulder width, for example—you are very stable. With your feet inside hip width, you are less stable, and you increase the stability challenge. This can also be applied when doing an exercise such as a cable standing antirotation press. When you perform it with the feet wide, it is easier, and when you bring your stance closer together it becomes more of a stability challenge to your torso musculature. This also applies when going from a regular squat to a single-leg squat. The single-leg squat on one foot has a narrower base; therefore the stability demands are increased.

Base of Support Points of Contact

Using the basic front plank as the example again, there are four points of contact on the ground—both of the forearms and both feet. If you pick up a foot or a hand, you now have three points of contact on the ground and thus the stability demands on the body are increased. We also refer to the points of contact as the amount of area in contact with the ground. We would classify exercises that move from supine (laying on the back) to standing as a progression within this principle because when you are standing, you have only two points of contact (the feet) on the ground versus when you are lying down, you have multiple points of contact and are very stable.

External Stability

External stability refers to the use of an implement or an object that will make you more unstable within the exercise. When you do a push-up on the floor, the ground provides a lot of stability because it doesn't move (except on occasion in California, of course). You can increase the amount of external instability by putting your hands (or feet) on a suspension training unit such as a TRX, or on a Swiss ball, while performing push-ups. Changing from a kettlebell single-arm overhead press to a kettlebell bottoms-up single-arm overhead press would be another example, because when you perform the press with the kettlebell turned upside down, you increase the stability challenge. Using a sandbag during various exercises is another example of how an unstable implement can vary the stability of an exercise.

Center of Mass Positioning

When you are in a standing position, your base of support is the middle of the foot. Our center of mass changes depending on where we place a load upon the body, and it also changes as we move. Since the external loads that we add to our bodies can be placed in a variety of positions, we can manipulate this to work toward our desired outcomes. Our system is most balanced (because of the influence of gravity) when our center of mass stays vertically aligned with our base of support. When we place an object's center of mass right in the middle of our foot (our base of support), such as in a kettlebell deadlift, we will also be in the most efficient position possible because our hips (the primary axis of rotation) will be horizontally closest to the kettlebell's center of mass.

An example of positioning our center of mass further from our base of support would be to go from a back squat to an overhead squat. The overhead squat isn't harder in terms of the amount of load being used because the load will actually be lighter, but it is more difficult to maintain the position while standing and moving. This occurs because the distance of the center of mass of the barbell and lifter system has been increased vertically from the base of support (in comparison to the back squat), and thus the stability demands have increased. If you want more loading you would choose the back squat, if you want more instability, you would go with the overhead squat.

Another way to increase muscular and stability demands is to place loads in a horizontal position relative to the base of support and the axis of rotation of the joints involved. An example of this would be to use an offset or asymmetrical load on the body such as in a kettlebell single-arm front squat. In a nutshell, whenever an object's center of mass is further from the base of support and the axis of rotation, the movement will be more challenging. You can manipulate this depending on the amount of stress that you want to impose on the body.

One final item to mention about this principle is that when you move the center of mass further from the axis of rotation you also increase the length of the lever arm. If you increase the distance lengthwise between two points of support while shifting the center of mass forward, you create an increased stability demand on the segments between the two end points. An example of this would be doing a roll-out with an ab wheel. This movement is typically performed on stationary knees with the hands moving forward as they hold the handles on the wheel. If you roll out as far as possible with your hands so that your body is almost parallel to the ground, you make the distance between your hands (or wheel) and knees greater than it would be if you stopped the wheel just under your shoulders. Thus, the muscular demands on your torso to stabilize the spine is higher due to the length of the lever that has been manipulated.

Range of Motion

A simple application of this principle is to modify the single-leg squat by squatting to the level of a soft box (as a depth marker) that is 18 inches (46 cm) high. You can progress and make it harder without increasing the external load by simply lowering the height of the box an inch at a time. This can also apply to a deadlift: In one phase we perform the deadlift from the floor, and in the next phase we deadlift from a two-inch (5 cm) deficit by standing on rubber mats. Increased range of motion can equate to more actual work being done.

Speed

Generally, we want to master slower speed movements before going faster. Most of the time, slow provides the foundation for fast. Deadlifts (which are "grindy" movements) should be mastered before moving to kettlebell swings (which are ballistic movements). Movement performance doesn't typically improve if you try to go faster before you can perform the movement well slowly. Speed can sometimes mask mistakes.

That said, this principle can be used to our advantage the other way around. Speed, or tempo (the cadence at which we perform our repetitions), can be used to make things feel harder. We can increase the relative intensity or the relative difficulty of an exercise without having to resort to increased external loading (sometimes going heavier is not the best option). Examples with general fitness clients are shown in chapter 7 and in some of the tool box workouts in chapter 9.

Movement Complexity

Basically, we want to master simple static movements before using more complex dynamic action movements. This can also apply to the number of joints involved in an

Tempo Refinement

Tempo refers to the speed at which a repetition or set of repetitions is to be performed. You can vary the rep speed to provide different training effects and you will see illustrations of this in our programming.

Arthur Jones of Nautilus fame was one of the first people to introduce rep speed or tempo to the exercise community. The late Charles Poliquin was the first to teach us about tempo, suggesting a three-digit formula to help coaches communicate how reps should be performed by their athletes (later refined to a four-digit formula). It's not hard to recognize that a bench press performed with a controlled eccentric lowering, a definite pause, and an explosive concentric lift is far different than a drop, bounce, and wiggle.

The three-digit formula is often written as 3-1-1 or just 311:

- The first number (3) refers to the eccentric or lowering portion of the lift.
- The second number (1) refers to the portion of the lift between the eccentric and concentric.
- The third number (1) refers to the concentric or lifting portion of the movement.

This makes sense if we perform a squat or bench press: a 3-second eccentric, pause for 1 second at the bottom, and then a 1-second concentric. But what about an exercise that begins with the concentric, like a chin-up? If the concentric portion of the exercise occurs first, we write it the same way for consistency, but we read it in reverse. The first number is always the eccentric and the third number is always the concentric. If there was a pause in this scenario it would occur after the concentric. In a chin-up example, you would do a 1-second concentric, pause at the top for 1 second, and then a 3-second eccentric. It is worth pointing out that in the past, a 1-second concentric portion meant it was performed as fast as possible. Currently, if we choose to use numbers to communicate that we want the concentric done as fast as possible, we replace the number 1 with the number 0 so that this is more clear.

In the past, we used this numerical system regularly to communicate tempo; however, we no longer use that method because it isn't an effective way to communicate how the rep should always be performed. That said, we still use a communication system and we still use the three-digit system on occasion when we want a very specific tempo used on an exercise.

To explain this further, telling a client to pause on the box or to hold the top of a back extension for a two-count is a form of tempo training prescription. Even the most vocal critic of tempo prescription would have to accept that doing front squats with a two-second pause at the bottom of each rep has an entirely different training effect than doing them without a pause. Clearly, rep speed can be used as a source of training variety and a potential varying stressor.

Most of the time, the concentric portion of most movements should be done as fast as possible (the load on the bar would dictate the speed), with the knowledge that on a set of higher reps (a set of 10 reps or more) you wouldn't go as fast as possible on the early reps.

We feel tempo variation should be used primarily to lengthen the eccentric component or to exploit or diminish the stretch–shortening cycle in the midpoint of the rep (the pause or transition time between the two actions). We occasionally prescribe a slower concentric when we want the client to focus on motor control issues, technical issues (such as falling forward on a back squat), deliberate and increased effort, and single-joint rehab movements.

If we say, "Lower it slowly, pause, and lift as fast as possible," or, "Do the entire rep as quickly as possible," we understand these commands as being two different training methods. Clearly, tempo does matter, but we have found that prescribing specific numbers to each phase of the lift isn't really necessary. Unless we use the traditional three-digit numerical system, we will prescribe the following shorthand and abbreviations to communicate tempo in our programs:

Tempo notation	Tempo definition
Slow	Slow tempo; controlled eccentric, definite pause, controlled concentric
Mod	Moderate tempo; controlled eccentric, definite pause, fast as possible concentric
— (em dash)	Normal tempo; controlled eccentric, no pause, fast as possible concentric
X	Fast tempo; fast eccentric, no pause, fast as possible concentric or explosive
Sec	Seconds; this is being used to communicate the parameters of the length of an isometric or static hold on an exercise. It is also used to communicate the length of an eccentric action on certain eccentric-only named exercises. In these cases, the other portions of the rep are not being considered in the execution of the movement
BR	Breaths; we use this to communicate number of breaths during a rep instead of using time. We often use this for mobility drills and the like
FE	Full exhale; this refers to a tempo where a full exhale is performed instead of a specific time count

Defining *controlled* can be difficult because one person's control is another's person's out of control. A solid test of control is, for example, the ability to stop on command during the eccentric phase of a bench press. Also, please note that the em dash (—) notation in the tempo column indicates a normal tempo or that the tempo of the exercise is implied by the nature of the exercise itself. An example of this would be a step up in which the previously listed tempo descriptors inadequately describe how to perform the movement.

exercise. Multijoint movements are more complex than simple single-joint movements because the more moving joints involved in an exercise, the more relatively complex a movement is; the less joints in motion, the less complexity. This concept of movement complexity can also apply to the progression from a split squat to a reverse lunge. When you perform a split squat, you are primarily performing a vertical level change as your center of mass moves up and down. When you progress to a reverse lunge, you are now moving your center of mass horizontally as well as vertically. Basically, in the reverse lunge you move down and back together, and then up and forward together, which is more complicated than only moving up and down as in a split squat.

Planes of Motion

Most training tends to be very sagittal-plane dominant with very little attention paid to training movement in the frontal and transverse planes of motion. How much training do you actually need to do in these planes of motion? To paraphrase Alwyn, "I can't tell you precisely how much you need to do, but I do know that zero is not enough."

The concept of functional training emphasizes the need to train the body beyond the sagittal plane because life and sport occur in all three planes of motion. The key point of this principle is to prioritize proficiency in the sagittal plane since we are most stable in this plane, and then progress to exercises that resist motion in the frontal and transverse planes, such as a single-leg RDL. Once proficient at resisting multiplanar forces, you then can progress to creating motion in the multiple planes of motion. As our colleague Josh Henkin, creator of the Ultimate Sandbag, quips, "Master the sagittal plane first, just don't stop there."

Progression and Regression
Within the Training Session Components

In chapter 1, we broke down our training plan to the beginning of the microcycle level and presented each of our daily training session components. Here are those components once again:

- RAMP (range of motion, activation, movement preparation)
- Core
- Power and elasticity or combination and rotation
- Strength and resistance training
- Energy system training
- Regeneration

We will now explain each component from an exercise standpoint, and then showcase the specific principle-based exercise progressions and regressions for several of the key movement patterns and for the specific exercises themselves. This will give you the tools to appropriately adjust a template to a client. Remember, exercise selection is the most individualized aspect of programming if goals and training age are relatively the same.

To minimize confusion when we use the terms *component* and *category* going forward, here are the definitions:

- *Components* differentiate the emphasis in the particular training session and create compartments within the training session itself.
- *Categories* classify and organize our exercises within each individual training session component.

Within several of the following training session components we are going to share our foundational exercise progressions. There are many types (or methods) of progressions and regressions for exercises, but it is crucial that these methods are based on principles, which is why we presented those principles first. As you review these exercise progressions, you will notice that there are various potential paths to take on some exercises in our categories. You can choose to pursue a load progression, or you can choose to increase the type of stability challenge, or one of the other principles. It is often helpful to plan for both, so we have provided some examples of each. Our purpose is to provide options, but also clarity, so that you have a reference point when it's necessary to make an exercise more challenging or less challenging on the spot.

Our goal is to simplify this classifying and categorization process. There are many different methods of categorizing movements and exercises that resonate with different coaches and organizations. We have found that our current classifying system works well, is relatively uncomplicated, and follows a solid rationale. We want it to be as unnecessarily complicated as possible without oversimplifying it to the point in which it doesn't make sense or it easily breaks down. Keep in mind that all methods of classifying and organizing have inherent trade-offs and are flawed to some degree. The key is having as few flaws as possible.

The reason we break down these sessions into categories and components is primarily for organizational purposes. Our brains tend to put things into compartments and by breaking down a training session, it allows the process to be taught. Sometimes it is difficult to make clear divisions between certain components and categories because it is hard to tell when one starts and another clearly stops. After all, when we finish the core component, have we really finished training our core? Of course not. Our core is going to be strongly involved in everything we do following the completion of that component! All training is core training just as all training is interconnected and the entire body itself is interconnected. Now, let's take a more detailed look at each of the training session components.

RAMP

We believe that most coaches and trainers (and clients, for that matter) would agree that a warm-up is important and worthwhile to begin a training session. Paradoxically, many of these same coaches and clients take this warm-up period lightly, and if they are going to skip something in their training session, the warm-up is what they tend to skip. We believe that this is a huge mistake.

The purpose of the warm-up period is to not only raise your body or core temperature. Old school warm-ups such as walking on a treadmill or riding on an exercise bike target the cardiovascular system and the lower body in primarily one plane of motion and in a very small range of motion. These activities do warm you up in the traditional sense, but it is not nearly as productive as it could be, and it is pretty boring to say the least. We can do better.

Instead of a warm-up, we prefer to call it RAMP which stands for range of motion, activation, and movement preparation. Many years ago, EXOS (formerly Athletes' Performance) founder Mark Verstegen and his team introduced the term *movement preparation* (MP) to the fitness coaching world in the groundbreaking book *Core Performance* (2004), and we fully adopted the term. This simple change in terminology immediately lends legitimacy to this component, and should be taken seriously. For our uses, we added to the movement preparation piece by adding RA (range of motion and activation) to the MP, making it an analogy that would stick with our clients. With a simple acronym, we give clarity to the real purpose of the warm-up.

In no particular order, the RAMP prepares the body in several ways:

- Potentially reduces targeted soft tissue tension and stiffness (e.g., self-massage with the foam roller or lacrosse ball)
- Primes muscle length and extensibility
- Primes the mobility and positioning of the joints by taking the body through multiple planes of movement, and provides some movement variability

- Elevates body and tissue temperature, and increases blood flow
- Prepares and excites the central nervous system to prepare the body for the demands of the workout and the movements and exercises that follow, such as squatting, hip-hinging, pulling, pushing, and rotational movements
- Provides an opportunity to ingrain quality motor skills in several movement patterns in a nonthreatening environment (simply put, it's a chance to practice and rehearse patterns before we start loading them)

A primary principle that we use with the RAMP is to start with exercises that are ground based (i.e., done on or near the floor), in-place, and relatively low intensity. We then progress to exercises that are done standing in-place, and advance to movements in which the client is moving across areas and covering ground (if space and logistics allow). These movements are more dynamic and integrated in nature. As you can see, intensity of effort and exercise complexity gradually ramps up as we move through this sequence. This tends to make the RAMP flow well and follow a nice logical sequence. It is analogous to starting a car and warming it up in place before you put it in gear, take off, and drive it hard.

The RAMP specifically contains the following elements.

Range of Motion and Activation

Range of motion and activation includes self-massage, stretching, or joint mobility exercises. Our RAMPs typically begin with the self-massage of three to four key areas or trouble spots with a foam roller, lacrosse ball, or other implements. We then perform a positional breathing drill to reset the top of our core (diaphragm) to face the bottom of our core (pelvic floor).

Next, we move to some ground-based mobility and activation drills that are focused on the thoracic spine (upper back), the hips in three dimensions, and the ankle. These areas tend to need increased mobility in most people. We may also activate several key muscles such as the hip stabilizers (the glute complex) and the scapular stabilizers (muscles around the shoulder blades).

Movement Preparation

We conclude with integrated dynamic stretching and movement patterns that take the body through fairly large excursions and multiple planes of motion. It may also conclude with some locomotive patterns such as marching, skipping patterns, or crawling. These activities serve to prime and prepare us for the movements that we are going to be performing in our forthcoming training session.

We can use this information to construct a basic RAMP template as shown in table 3.2. Keep in mind that this template is not set in stone. It is an outline that can be modified when warranted, but these are often the qualities that we want to address.

In terms of the dosages and timing constraints, we typically try to cap the RAMP at a maximum of 10 to 15 minutes (not including the 3 to 5 minutes spent on self-massage). We can often use movements that combine several of the elements together to make the RAMP as time efficient as possible, but from a programming standpoint, these boxes should generally be checked off unless it is warranted not to.

Core

This word may be the most overused and misunderstood term in all of the fitness industry. The very mention of it can make some fitness authorities shudder in dis-

Table 3.2 Basic RAMP Template

RAMP element	Comments
Self-massage	3-4 targeted spots (no more than 3-5 min spent on this prework-out).
Positional breathing reset	Choose 1 exercise emphasizing diaphragmatic breathing and rib and pelvis positioning.
Hip stretch and activation	Target hip extension mobility, hip adduction mobility, and hip rotation mobility.
T-spine mobilization and activation	Target thoracic spine mobility in extension and rotation, scapular stabilization.
Ankle mobilization	Target ankle dorsiflexion.
Standing hip activation	Banded work or single-leg stance exercises
Combination	Integrated movement with one hip in flexion and one hip in extension. Often done in closed-chain positions to work on scapular stabilization.
Priming and patterning (single-leg stance hip hinge)	Typically, a bodyweight single-leg RDL or patterning drill.
Priming and patterning (asymmetrical stance squat and lunge)	1-2 lunge variations (make sure one is multiplanar as warranted).
Priming and patterning (squat)	Symmetrical-stance squat patterning and mobility drill.
Movement skills (optional)	Pick 2-3 locomotive patterns such as skipping or crawling.
Neural activation (optional)	Pick 1 neural activation exercise such as a high-frequency, low-amplitude side-to-side jump performed for a short duration.

Note: Light gray denotes range of motion and activation sections, and dark gray denotes movement preparation sections.

gust. Conversely, the word can make our clients smile ear to ear when then learn that something is a core exercise. We use the term *core* as a component for our direct or targeted torso training. It may not be the best term, but it is the most familiar, so we use it for communication purposes with our clients and other coaches. This is one of those concessions to the mainstream because core is such a commonly accepted term.

Even though it's a common term, what is the core exactly? This is a truly loaded question and we can go down a massive rabbit hole to answer it. For the sake of brevity, we consider the core to be comprised of the muscles that act on the pelvis, the lumbar spine, and the rib cage. These muscles are not limited to, but include the following:

- diaphragm
- rectus abdominus
- erector spinae
- external and internal obliques
- transverse abdominis
- pelvic floor
- quadratus lumborum
- multifidi
- glutes, hamstrings, and hip rotators
- latissimus dorsi

It's incredibly helpful to think of the core as a cannister. In a nutshell, the goal of most core exercises is to keep the top of the core cannister (the diaphragm) facing the bottom of the cannister (the pelvic floor) while resisting unwanted movement.

Core Evolutions and Research

The core component of our training sessions is the one that has undergone the most rapid evolutions and changes over the past 10 to 15 years. Many of our current ideas on core training have been strongly influenced and shaped by the teachings of Gray Cook, Stuart McGill, Mike Boyle, and Shirley Sahrmann. Over the past three to five years, Josh Henkin, the creator of the Ultimate Sandbag, has had a profound impact on how we approach core training (2019). The sandbag has become an integral tool due its unique ability to create cross-linking of the body's fascial chains.

These fitness experts emphasize that the primary function of our core is to resist unwanted motion (rather than creating extraneous movement in the lumbar spine in particular) and to tie the upper and lower quadrants of body together minimizing any potential "leaks." Investigate the work of these authors for further information on this expansive topic.

Let's get something out of the way: It is a myth that you need to do crunches to work the abs. There have been numerous studies declaring that bridges and planks are safer than abdominal crunches (see Stuart McGill's work), but many coaches still have clients doing large numbers of crunches because they feel the benefit is worth the risk.

However, one study concluded that an Ab Slide device elicited the greatest EMG activity for the abdominal muscles and the least for the rectus femoris (Youdas et al. 2008). Another study compared infomercial ab training devices to crunches and sit ups. The conclusions in this study were that the Ab Slide and Torso Track were the most effective exercises in activating abdominal and upper extremity muscles while minimizing low back and rectus femoris (hip flexion) activity (Escamilla et al. 2006).

While both of these studies looked at infomercial devices, which immediately turns most of us off, don't let that mislead you. Both are essentially abdominal roll-outs or planks in which there is no flexion or actual movement of the spine, and the activation is due to stabilization demands. You don't need an infomercial product to reproduce that movement. In other words, an ab roll-out exercise may be more effective at activating the rectus abdominus than crunches or sit-ups. So not only are the planks and roll-outs a safer option, they could actually be a superior choice.

Another interesting study indicated that a group performing only core stabilization exercises (no sit-ups) had a slightly improved performance during sit-up testing compared to a group that trained the actual sit-up (Childs et al. 2009). So it's pretty clear based upon the evidence that it is a win-win situation. Core stability training is the key to building successful athletes (we consider all of our clients to be athletes). Most coaches working with competitive athletes would also like them to perform more core stability exercises. It's that important. For general population clients it's typically their greatest weakness and main limiting factor (a large majority of beginners are unable to perform even a single push-up).

Core Priority

The logic that you should always train the core at the end of a session has never made much sense to us. The argument is that if you intensely train the core at the beginning of the workout, you risk fatiguing it, and having that fatigue negatively affect the rest of the session. This is a fair argument, but is it true? Since the core is commonly one of the weakest areas for most individuals, then why not give it the attention it deserves and train it as a priority? If it is your weakest area, then it should be trained first. We strongly adhere to the principle that whatever gets trained first gets the most benefit.

When we look at squatting, the abs don't work concentrically coming out of a squat, so we're not concerned if an athlete performed a front plank for 30 to 45 seconds in the core section component prior to executing a squat in the strength section component. How much fatigue is actually generated here? How long would the fatigue last? Does it impact the squat performance and safety? We think it is critical to examine these questions.

Interestingly, as Coach Mike Boyle mentions in the second edition of his book *Functional Training for Sports* (2016), since so many of our core exercises are more isometric in nature, they may actually be "upregulating" muscles more so than they would be fatiguing them. This is yet another potential reason to do them first.

If it's important and it's a priority, then let's prioritize it and put it at the beginning!

Core Categories

We currently categorize our core exercises in a similar manner to several of our esteemed colleagues. Most notably, we use many of the same terms that coach Mike Boyle does in his aforementioned book.

We look at direct core training as being primarily composed of the following elements:

- *Antiextension (AE):* Resisting excessive extension of the lumbar spine.
- *Antirotation (AR):* Resisting rotation of the lumbar spine. It also involves some antiextension characteristics by nature.
- *Antilateral flexion (AF):* Resisting lateral flexion of the lumbar spine.
- *Hip flexion (HF):* Flexion of the hip joint with a stable lumbar spine.

It is important to note that many exercises that we classify as either antiextension or antirotation have elements of both and exist on another type of continuum between pure antiextension and pure antirotation (see figure 3.2). As you move to the right on the continuum, you are resisting rotation at the lumbar spine, and at the same time, resisting extension during various exercises. When classifying exercises, you have to decide on a category even though the lines may be blurry at times. For us, once the demands of rotary stability or extension are introduced to an appreciable amount, we place it toward the right or left side of the continuum (represented by vertical line) for the sake of making programming choices.

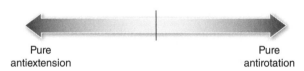

Pure antiextension

Pure antirotation

Figure 3.2 Core exercise antiextension to antirotation continuum.

When we examine our exercises closely, we can subclassify the type of stability we are using in some of our categories previously discussed. (This falls into principle 8 in our list of progression and regression principles: movement complexity.) The stability of the core exercises in each category can be subclassified as follows:

- *Static stabilization:* No motion occurring in any of the limbs of the body while the spine is stable; static hip joint and static shoulder joint (e.g., a front plank).
- *Dynamic stabilization:* The hip joint is stable while the shoulder joint moves (e.g., a cable bar half-kneeling chop) or the shoulder joint is stable while the hip joint moves (e.g., a suspension trainer prone jackknife).
- *Integrated stabilization:* Dynamic motion that occurs about the shoulders and hips with a relatively stable lumbar spine. This is how we look at rotational exercises and most complex movement in general. We still view these exercises as core exercises to an extent, but placing them into our combination component tends to be a better fit.

ıg *Core Exercises*

ry entry point into the core category from an exercise standpoint is the front
the lowly and mundane front plank. As fundamental as it is, it is often
nd quickly glossed over. TRX director of programming Chris Frankel and
ach Dan John have written and spoken extensively about the virtues of
position. They have observed that just about everything we do in the gym
is a plank. Therefore, this fundamental position of our torso can be observed in many
primal movements and various exercises.

Our colleague and StrongFirst's director of education Brett Jones likens good exercise
form to being akin to a Sasquatch sighting: "Often talked about, rarely seen." This
is how we feel about good form on the front plank and the side plank in particular.
Bottom line, we are militant about proper plank position; as unsexy as it may seem, a
properly performed plank of any kind can be a real eye-opener to our clients. It may
not look like much is happening on the outside, but there is a lot going on in the inside
in regard to the muscular demands if it is performed to the highest standards.

Here's how we subcategorize the core component: First, figure 3.3 illustrates the
primary category and subcategories; then tables 3.3 through 3.8 show our actual base
exercise progressions moving from easiest to hardest (for example, progression number
1 would be easiest and progression number 3 would be harder). Please refer to the
How Progressions and Regressions Work sidebar on page 44 for more information
on how to apply these tables in practice. We also provide descriptions and photos of
less-common exercises at the end of the chapter.

Power and Elasticity or Combination and Rotation

Power and elasticity or combination and rotation are technically two separate components, but one or the other will be performed right after the core component and
before our main resistance training depending on training session, the client's goal, and

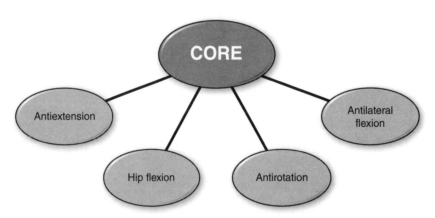

Figure 3.3 Core subcategories.

Table 3.3 Core: Antiextension Progressions 1

Progression		Exercise
1 Easier	↑	Front plank (use incline front plank if further regression is needed)
2		Suspension trainer front plank (feet in suspension trainer)
3		Suspension trainer body saw (can use slide board as an alternative)
4		Swiss ball fallout
5		Suspension trainer kneeling fallout
6 Harder	↓	Wheel kneeling roll-out

Table 3.4 Core: Antiextension Progressions 2

Progression		Exercise
1 Easier	↑	Sandbag dead bug with alternating 90° heel touch (use band if sandbag is not available)
2		Sandbag full-dead bug with alternating leg reach
3		Sandbag full-dead bug with alternating arm turn
4		Sandbag full-dead bug with alternating arm reach
5		Hollow isometric hold
6 Harder	↓	Hollow rocking

Table 3.5 Core: Hip Flexion Progressions

Progressions		Exercise
1 Easier	↑	Sandbag unsupported leg-lowering (alternating)
2		Suspension trainer prone jackknife
3		Suspension trainer mountain climber
4		Suspension trainer prone pike
5		Hanging knee raise
6		Eccentric-only hanging leg raise
7 Harder	↓	Hanging leg raise

Table 3.6 Core: Antirotation Progressions 1

Progressions		Exercise
1 Easier	↑	Sandbag quadruped birddog isometric hold (alternating)
2		Sandbag quadruped birddog lateral drag
3		Sandbag quadruped bear isometric hold (alternating)
4		Sandbag quadruped bear lateral drag
5		Sandbag tall-plank lateral isometric hold (alternating)
6 Harder	↓	Sandbag tall-plank lateral drag

Table 3.7 Core: Antirotation Progressions 2

Progressions		Exercise
1 Easier	↑	Cable kneeling antirotation press (use band if cable machine is not available)
2		Cable half-kneeling antirotation press
3		Cable bar kneeling chop or lift
4		Cable bar half-kneeling chop or lift
5		Cable standing antirotation press + overhead raise
6 Harder	↓	Standing antirotation variations: Once beyond progression 5, there are several options available to the programmer. The previous levels serve as a foundational prerequisite prior to moving to other antirotation variations.

Table 3.8 Core: Antilateral Flexion Progressions

Progressions		Exercise
1 Easier	↑	Sandbag side plank (from knees)
2		Side plank
3		Suspension trainer side plank
4		Side plank + cable single-arm row
5		Kettlebell single-arm farmer's walk (use dumbbell if kettlebell is not available)
6		Kettlebell single-arm bottoms-up rack walk
7 Harder	↓	Kettlebell single-arm waiter's walk

the client's phase. Power exercises are movements that require the system to produce force in a short period of time. This component is done in the freshest state immediately after the core training piece to display and produce as much power as possible. Power training is critical for competitive athletes to enhance sport performance, but it is also critical for everyone in some form. As one ages, there is a gradual decline in lean body mass and an even sharper decline in power development.

Therefore, there must be high priority in attenuating the decline of power production as one ages. This is especially important for the aging members of the gym to enhance functional capacity later in life. We use the term *elasticity* to refer to plyometric and jumping-type activities. Combination movements refer to exercises that combine movement patterns together in some way. Rotation movements are closely related to our combination exercises because rotation is actually combined movement patterns performed in the transverse plane. Many of our integrated core exercises mentioned earlier can be placed in this component as well. We will dive into more specific exercise details of this component when we provide specific programming examples later in the book.

Strength and Resistance Training

Strength and resistance training is the meat and potatoes for most goals. Alwyn likens strength training to being a cheat code in athletics. *Cheat code* meaning that being as strong as possible gives one an unfair but completely legal advantage over others if all else is equal.

Strength and Resistance Training Categories

The way we categorize our movement patterns and exercises within this component (and all the other training session components) is constantly evolving. We are truly driven by the idea that there must be a better way. As such, how we currently classify and categorize the resistance training component for our training sessions is slightly different than what you may have seen in the past if you are familiar with our previous materials. We always reserve the right to improve and to get better, so we hope you, the reader, will understand and appreciate that fact.

That said, the evolution of all this is aptly stated with a quote commonly attributed to noted physical therapist Gary Gray: "If we train movement, muscles will never be forgotten. If we train muscles, movement is sure to be forgotten." One key principle of our system of training and programming is to focus on exercise selection around movements—*not* muscle groups. Gray's quote really encapsulates this principle. To build muscle (or even maintain it) we have to work the muscle. And to build muscle everywhere, we have to work every muscle in the body.

There are over 600 muscles in the body, so you can already see the problem with the bodybuilding "isolation" approach. We have to work the muscles in groups. Traditionally, bodybuilders have used muscle groups or body part splits. Powerlifters have typically gravitated towards a lift-specific split (bench, squat, and deadlift) and then further divided their workouts into upper- and lower-body routines (because of the overlap). Olympic lifters use total body workouts as do most athletes.

Instead of copying what other sports do, let's look at what *the body* does. If we break down everything that the body can do, we come up with a plethora of activities such as running, jumping, rotating, climbing, throwing, crawling, bending, pushing, kicking, and pulling. Recall that when we break it down, the body can only do six movements: squat, lunge, bend, push, pull, and twist.

As mentioned previously in chapter 2, this was first discovered by Richard Schmidt in his book *Motor Learning and Performance* (1991) who proposed that the brain stores key movements in a relative timing sequence that is easily modified in both velocity and amplitude to become other movements. A leg press machine is essentially a modified squat (albeit using less total muscle). Climbing stairs is a combination of squatting and lunging. Throwing the javelin is really just a lunge, twist, and push performed in a series (as is a punch). Just about every single athletic activity can be broken down into those movements. To train everything— all we really need to do is target those six movements. That doesn't mean we need to do all six movements at every single workout, or even in every phase of the program; it means we have to recognize what the body *does*, and train those movements and therefore, those muscles.

These patterns are still the basis for what we continue to do today because the body and brain recognize these movements and works in terms of movements not muscles. We continue to use all of these primal patterns in the structure of our training sessions; we just put them in different places now. These patterns and their combinations are natural to the body, and that is how we prefer to think about our training. Don't get us wrong, we love muscles, but one glance at Thomas Myers' *Anatomy Trains* book or a quick trip to the famous Body World's traveling anatomy exhibit, and you realize that the body is not a collection of parts, but is very much an integrated and connected system.

Classifying Strength and Resistance Exercises

Several years ago we reclassified some elements of the strength and resistance component so that it matched up with the Functional Movement Screen (see chapter 2). We had previously used the single-leg stance as a stand-alone category for a movement pattern, but on reexamination realized that the single-leg stance is simply a foot position, not a movement pattern, so it didn't make sense to classify it as stand-alone movement pattern. Single-leg stance is now included in both the hip hinge and squat subcategories. You will probably also note that the lunge is not listed in our movement pattern categorization. We now subcategorize our primary four movement patterns in this component by foot position or body position. So, our lunge actually fits into the squat category because the hips move up and down in a level change in an asymmetrical foot position or split stance.

Also, some coaches use upper- and lower-push and upper- and lower-pull to classify their movement patterns, but while we feel that push and pull works well for the upper body, it does not work as well as the squat and hinge do for the lower body. Dan John, who popularized the goblet squat, also developed the squat–hinge continuum (a continuum that refers to the degree of how much the hips displace back versus down in squatting and hip-hinging exercises) referred to in the book *Deadlift Dynamite* by Pavel Tsatsouline and Andy Bolton (2012). Ultimately, this is largely semantics and all attempts to classify movement patterns are going to have flaws on some level, but the classification system that we are currently using seems to work very well and makes sense to us and to our coaches.

The primary movement pattern categories that we use are squat, hip hinge, push, and pull. These primary movements are further subcategorized by foot position or body ion. Figure 3.4 illustrates the primary category and subcategories; then tables 3.9 gh 3.19 show the base exercise progressions moving from easiest to hardest (for ple, progression number 1 would be easiest and progression number 3 would be harder). Please refer to the How Progressions and Regressions Work sidebar at the end of this chapter for more information on how to apply these tables in practice. We will also provide descriptions and photos of less-common exercises at the end of the chapter.

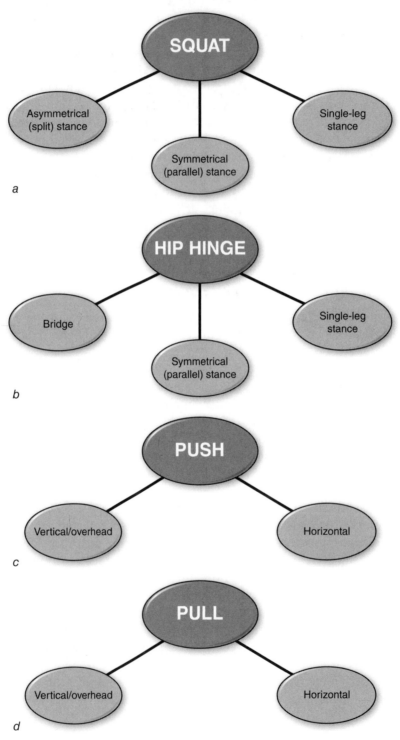

Figure 3.4 Squat *(a)*, hip hinge *(b)*, push *(c)*, and pull *(d)* subcategories.

Table 3.9   Squat: Asymmetrical (Split) Stance Progressions

Progressions		Exercise
1 Easier	↑	Assisted bottoms-up split squat → bodyweight split squat
2		Goblet split squat → two-dumbbell split squat
3		Goblet rear-foot-elevated split squat → two-dumbbell rear-foot-elevated split squat
4		Goblet reverse lunge → two-dumbbell reverse lunge
5		Two-dumbbell forward lunge *or* two-dumbbell walking lunge
6 Harder	↓	Lateral lunge and cross-behind lunge

Table 3.10   Squat: Symmetrical (Parallel) Stance Progressions

Progressions		Exercise
1 Easier	↑	Assisted squat or bodyweight box squat
2		Goblet squat
3		Two-kettlebell front squat
4		Barbell front squat
5 Harder	↓	Barbell back squat

Table 3.11   Squat: Single-Leg Stance Progressions

Progressions		Exercise
1 Easier	↑	Bodyweight step-up (progress or regress ROM as needed)
2		Goblet step-up
3		Goblet sprinter step-up
4		Single-leg skater squat
5		Single-leg squat to box
6 Harder	↓	Single-leg squat from box

Table 3.12   Hip Hinge: Symmetrical (Parallel) Stance Bridge Progressions

Progressions		Exercise
1 Easier	↑	Double-leg hip bridge
2		Shoulder-elevated hip bridge
3		Swiss ball eccentric-only supine hip extension leg curl (use a suspension trainer as an alternative)
4		Swiss ball supine hip extension leg curl
5		Slider eccentric-only supine hip extension leg curl
6 Harder	↓	Slider supine hip extension leg curl

Table 3.13   Hip Hinge: Symmetrical (Parallel) Stance Progressions

Progressions		Exercise
1 Easier	↑	Prisoner bodyweight Romanian deadlift
2		Kettlebell deadlift
3		High hex bar deadlift *or* Romanian deadlift
4		Block deadlift
5		Deadlift
6 Harder	↓	Deficit deadlift *or* snatch- (wide-) grip deadlift

Table 3.14 Hip Hinge: Single-Leg Stance Progressions

Progressions		Exercise
1 Easier	↑	Assisted *or* bodyweight single-leg Romanian deadlift
2		One-dumbbell block single-leg deadlift *or* one-dumbbell staggered-stance Romanian deadlift *or* one-dumbbell slider single-leg Romanian deadlift
3		One-dumbbell single-leg Romanian deadlift
4		Two-dumbbell single-leg Romanian deadlift
5 Harder	↓	Barbell single-leg Romanian deadlift

Table 3.15 Push: Vertical/Overhead Progressions

Progressions		Exercise
1 Easier	↑	Kettlebell kneeling or half-kneeling single-arm overhead press (use dumbbell if kettlebell not available; can use landmine instead of kettlebell if client is not cleared to go overhead)
2		Kettlebell half-kneeling single-arm overhead press
3		Two-kettlebell overhead press
4		Kettlebell alternating overhead press
5		Barbell overhead press
6 Harder	↓	Barbell push press

Table 3.16 Push: Horizontal (Push-up) Progressions

Progressions		Exercise
1 Easier	↑	Push-up (use incline as further regression if needed)
2		Resisted or feet-elevated push-up
3		Suspension trainer push-up
4		Single-leg push-up
5		T-push-up
6 Harder	↓	Multiple push-up variations: Once beyond progression 5, there are several options available to the programmer. The previous levels serve as a foundational prerequisite prior to moving to other push-up variations.

Table 3.17 Push: Horizontal (Bench Press) Progressions

Progressions		Exercise
1 Easier	↑	Dumbbell single-arm bench press
2		Dumbbell bench press
3		Dumbbell alternating bench press or barbell bench press
4		Dumbbell single-arm bench press on half-bench or other bench press variations
5 Harder	↓	Cable split-stance single-arm forward press

Table 3.18   Pull: Vertical/Overhead (Chin-up) Progressions

Progressions	Exercise
1 Easier ↑	Kneeling or half-kneeling pulldowns (can use various grips; we often use neutral grip because it tends to be very shoulder friendly)
2	Suspension trainer inverted neutral-grip row (this is a horizontal row but we use it to bridge the gap from pulldown to chin-up)
3	Top of chin-up isometric hold *or* band-assisted chin-up
4	Eccentric-only chin-up
5	Chin-up
6	Neutral-grip pull-up
7 Harder ↓	Pull-up

Table 3.19   Pull: Horizontal (Row) Progressions

Progressions	Exercise
1 Easier ↑	Cable half-kneeling single-arm row
2	Cable single-arm neutral-grip row *or* cable standing row
3	Dumbbell bench row *or* dumbbell three-point row *or* cable seated neutral-grip row
4	Suspension trainer inverted neutral-grip row
5	Dumbbell two-point single-leg neutral-grip row
6 Harder ↓	Barbell overhand-grip dead row

Energy System Training

In this component of our training session we create specific metabolic conditioning work for our clients if it follows the resistance training session. This is something that will be very dependent on the client's goals and available training time. At our gym we often prescribe it to be performed on a different day. The specific reasons for this will be expanded on in the programming session as warranted.

Regeneration

Our final component is regeneration. Remember this mantra, "You don't get better by training, you get better by recovering from training." At our gym the most common postworkout method is to have our clients do a breathing drill before they have post-workout nutrition.

This breathing drill is the cool down and it tones down the client by getting the nervous system back into a parasympathetic (rest and digest) state after being in a sympathetic state (fight or flight) during the training session. This gets them back on the road to recovery after the training session. The regeneration component can also take the form of some light static stretching that focuses on breathing, or soft tissue or self-massage work on problematic areas. We provide examples of how to design the breathing drill in later chapters.

How Progressions and Regressions Work

If you are implementing a program and find that an exercise is not an appropriate fit for a client (they are currently over- or underqualified for it), you would refer to the table and select the more appropriate exercise. You simply make sure that the exercise chosen within a movement pattern for a particular client matches the client's current ability level. If it doesn't, you need to move it up or down a level. Sometimes you only need to make sure the correct load is being applied. If an exercise is too easy or too hard it often stems from using the wrong weight. If it is not a load issue, an exercise change may be warranted.

We have developed a coaching algorithm (see figure 3.5) to show how the decision-making process works so that it can be taught to others:

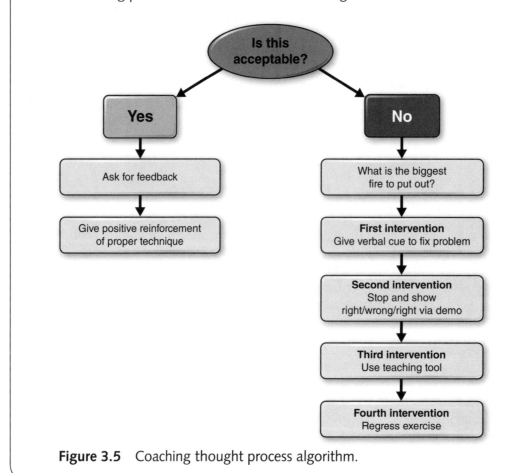

Figure 3.5 Coaching thought process algorithm.

Now you have a fundamental understanding of the thought processes and principles behind how we develop and select exercise progressions and regressions in several of the key components that make up a training session. We encourage you to use them in practice with your clients. As you gain experience and knowledge, we encourage you to refine them and create progressions and regressions that are unique to your own skill set. You can even use your own exercise nomenclature, but we strongly recommend consistency. Most importantly, be sure that your exercise progressions and regressions are based on a sound set of principles such as the nine we previously listed.

SELECT CORE EXERCISES

SUSPENSION TRAINER BODY SAW

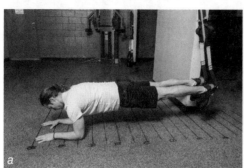 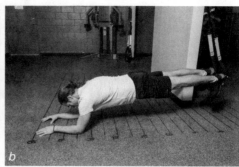

Setup and Performance

- Adjust the bottom of the foot straps so that they hang at midshin. Place feet in straps so that they are even when you are facing the ground.
- Get into a front plank position with the elbows stacked directly under the shoulder joints and the forearms parallel to each other.
- Maintain the plank position while pushing the body away from the shoulders. Pull back into the starting position with the shoulders stacked over elbows or very slightly in front of them.

Key Performance Points

- Keep the face pushed away from the ground and the neck in a neutral position.
- This exercise should not be felt in the lumbar spine.
- Keep full body tension while moving forward and backward to maintain the core cannister position.

SWISS BALL FALLOUTS

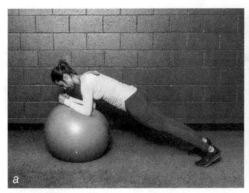 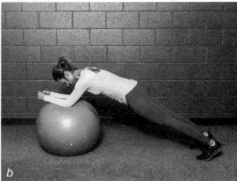

Setup and Performance

- Begin in a plank position with the forearms and elbows in the center of the Swiss ball. The feet will be no more than hip-width apart.
- Maintain a plank position while sliding the elbows and forearms forward, rolling the Swiss ball forward. Pull the elbows back toward the body, returning to the starting position.
- This exercise is similar but opposite to the body saw. In this exercise, the feet are planted and remain stationary while the forearms move, whereas in the body saw it is the reverse.

Key Performance Points

- Keep the face pushed away from the ground and the neck in a neutral position.
- Keep full body tension throughout entire movement. Squeeze the glutes, tighten the quads, and push the floor away with the feet.
- Keep the ribs and hips together as you move the elbows forward. This is an exercise that should not be felt in the lumbar spine.

SANDBAG FULL DEAD BUG
WITH ALTERNATING LEG REACH

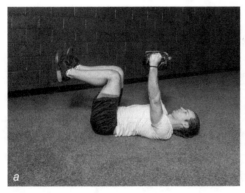 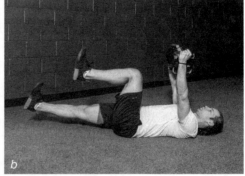

Setup and Performance

- Lie on the back and bring the legs up into a 90-degree hip- and knee-bend position.
- Hold the sandbag by the outside handles over your chest with the wrist straight and fully extended arms.
- Pull the handles of the bag apart and bring the ribs down to slightly press the low back into the floor.
- Maintaining tension, extend one leg so that it hovers slightly off the ground. Fully exhale at this position. Return to the starting position and repeat on the other side.

Key Performance Points

- Be sure to pull the handles of the sandbag apart while extending the leg. This will help create and maintain top-down body tension and pelvic stability. Prevent the bag from sagging.
- Reset the tension between each rep.

HOLLOW ROCKING

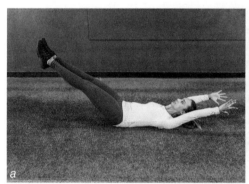 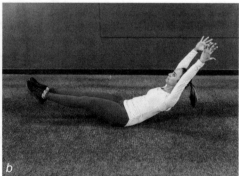

Setup and Performance

- Start by lying on your back. Pull the bottom of the ribs toward the bony points of the top of the pelvis. Lift the legs off the floor and extend the arms overhead. Keep the legs straight and the toes pointed. Your body will be in a slight curve, resembling a banana shape. In this position you begin to rock. Imagine you are rocking on the ground like a rocking chair.

Key Performance Points

- The hollow position and name comes to us from gymnastics. It's not the old idea of sucking in the abs. It is locking the rib cage down to the pelvis and maintaining that distance when forces are trying to pull it apart.
- The key to this exercise is creating tension from the tips of the toes through the fingertips.
- Maintain the set distance between the rib cage and pelvis. They must remain "tied" together as you rock.

SUSPENSION TRAINER PRONE PIKE

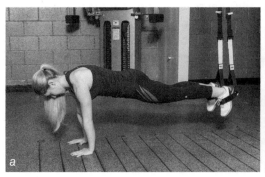 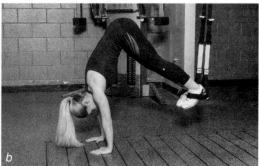

Setup and Performance

- Adjust the bottom of the foot straps so that they hang at midshin.
- Place the foot straps on the feet and get into a tall plank position with hands under the shoulders and the feet positioned under the anchor point.
- Keeping the legs straight and the feet together, bend at the hip and lift the hips as high as possible while keeping the spine stable.

Key Performance Points

- Keep the arms straight and feet dorsiflexed (shoelaces pulled towards shins).
- Keep the neck in neutral position; do not "chicken neck."

SANDBAG QUADRUPED BIRDDOG LATERAL DRAG

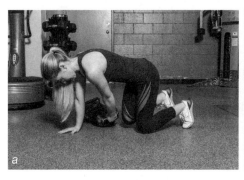 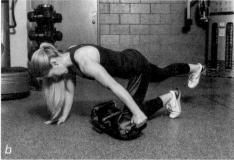

Setup and Performance

- Start on the hands and knees, the knees under the hips and the hands under the shoulders, both the hands and knees are about shoulder-width apart. The toes are tucked under.
- Grip the floor with your hands. The sandbag will start on one side of the body.
- Grab the outside handle of the sandbag with the opposite side hand (i.e., the bag is on the left side of your body and you grab it with the right hand, dragging the bag from left to right) as you pick up the knee diagonal to this hand.

- The thumb of the hand pulling the bag will point forward. As you pull the bag underneath you, extend the leg opposite to the hand dragging away from you. This will leave you with two points of contact on the ground and one hand on the sandbag. Once the bag is pulled as far as you can without losing position, switch hands and legs and go back in the other direction.

Key Performance Points

- Maintain a stable pelvis while the bag is moving and the point of stability from the leg is removed.
- When the bag is being pulled, keep it low, pulling it under the stomach, just slightly in front of the belly button. It should be closer to the thighs than it is to the arms.
- Pull slowly! Keep the bag even and flat on the ground while dragging will help with this.

SANDBAG TALL-PLANK LATERAL DRAG

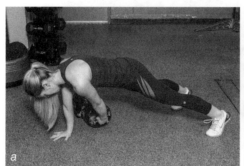 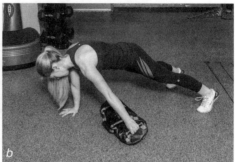

Setup and Performance

- Start in a typical push-up position with the hands under the shoulders and the legs straight.
- Set the feet wider than shoulder-width and position the bag off to one side of the body.
- Pick up one hand while keeping the hips stable and pull the bag across to the opposite side, keeping the bag slightly in front of the belly button.

Key Performance Points

- Maintain a stable pelvis while the bag is moving.
- Pull slowly! Keeping the bag even and flat on the ground as you drag it will help with this.
- Keep the pulling arm straight and the shoulder away from the ear as the bag is pulled.
- If the hips are turning, widen the feet.

CABLE BAR KNEELING CHOP

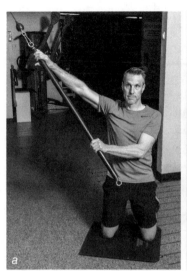 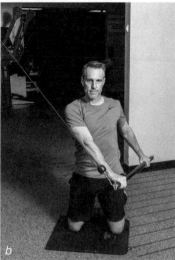

Setup and Performance

- Attach a cable bar or a long rope to an adjustable cable machine with a high pulley that is set to approximately head height when standing.
- Get into a tall kneeling position (both knees down) next to the machine and turn perpendicular to the pulley.
- Use an overhand grip on the cable bar.
- Pull the bar across the body keeping the bar close to the torso, and then move both arms out at the bottom, moving the cable in a diagonal line.

Key Performance Points

- Be sure to keep the torso stacked through the whole movement. Keep the rib cage stacked over the hips. Think of this as a tall-kneeling plank.
- There will be some rotation and motion through the upper back and the shoulders but keep the hips static.

CABLE STANDING ANTIROTATION PRESS + OVERHEAD RAISE

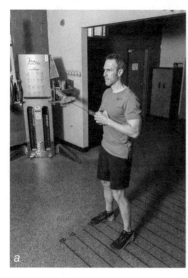 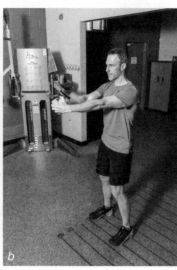 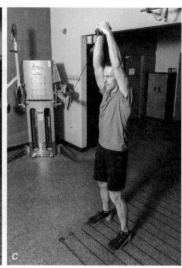

Setup and Performance

- Attach a handle to the cable machine with the pulley set to about midchest height.
- Set the feet shoulder-width apart or slightly narrower.
- Grab the machine handle with the outside hand and place the other hand on top. Bring the handle to the lower sternum.
- Press out in line with the handle until the arms are fully extended and then raise the handle overhead keeping the handle lined up with the middle of the body throughout.
- Reverse the movement and return to the starting position and repeat.

Key Performance Points

- Imagine that the handle is like a saw cutting the body into an equal left and right half.
- Keep the body stable while the arms are moving.

SUSPENSION TRAINER SIDE PLANK

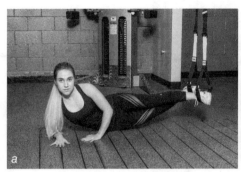 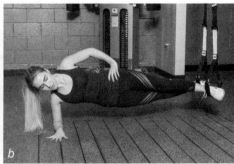

Setup and Performance

- Adjust the bottom of the foot straps so that they hang at midshin.
- Lie on your side and place the foot straps on the feet and get into a side plank position.
- The top leg will be in front and the bottom leg will be directly behind it with the front heel touching the back toe.
- The body will be in a straight line from the head to the top-leg heel.
- Hold for the designated time and repeat as prescribed.

Key Performance Points

- Push through on the ground with the forearm before lifting the hips up into a side plank.
- Keep the elbow stacked under the shoulder.
- Make sure the feet are steady in the suspension trainer before moving the hips off the floor.

KETTLEBELL SINGLE-ARM WAITER'S WALK

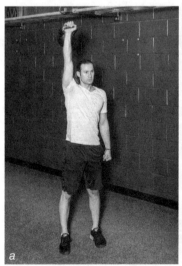 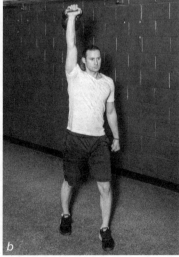

Setup and Performance

- Press an appropriately weighted kettlebell overhead with the arm completely straight and vertical as viewed from the front and back.
- Walk with the kettlebell overhead for the designated distance holding the kettlebell in the proper position.
- Bring the kettlebell down efficiently and repeat on the opposite side.

Key Performance Points

- Keep the shoulder away from the ear.
- Keep the opposite arm fairly close the side to prevent it from becoming a counterweight.

SELECT STRENGTH AND RESISTANCE EXERCISES

TWO-KETTLEBELL FRONT SQUAT

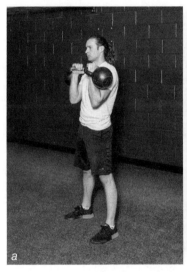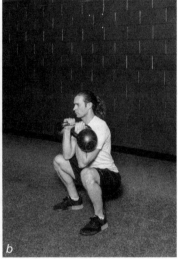

Setup and Performance

- Situate two kettlebells into a front rack position. You can do this by cleaning the kettlebells or by having someone hand you a bell once you have one in position.
- The kettlebells will rest on the outside of the forearms. The forearms will be vertical.
- Set the feet about shoulder-width apart with the toes turned out slightly. Stand tall.
- Take a deep breath and squat down between the feet so that tops of the thighs are below parallel to the floor.
- Return to the starting position and repeat.

Key Performance Points

- Be sure the knees track in line with the toes.
- Look straight ahead.
- "Screw" the feet into the floor to create tension and stability.
- Pull the kettlebells into the body to make them feel as if they are a part of the body.

ASSISTED BOTTOMS-UP SPLIT SQUAT

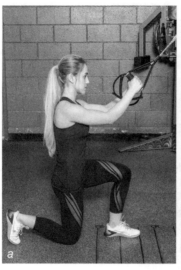 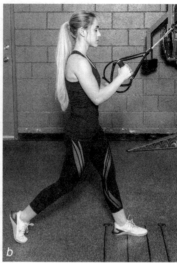

Setup and Performance

- Start on the floor holding onto a suspension trainer and get into a half-kneeling position with the front knee and the hip set close to a 90-degree angle (the front shin angle can be slightly forward). When the back knee is on the floor it will also be set close to a 90-degree angle.
- Create tension by bracing the core and leveling out the pelvis side to side and from the front to back.
- Using the suspension trainer as much or as little as needed, stand up into the top of a split squat position.
- Lower back down to the floor, reset, and repeat.

Key Performance Points

- Digging in the back toe and "turning up the belt buckle" to level the pelvis will help teach the proper position at the bottom, the most challenging portion of the movement. This is also a great way to determine stance length and width when performing other types of split squats.
- After each rep, reset completely on the ground with a dead stop.
- Ensure that the back knee, hip, and shoulder are stacked and in-line at the bottom.
- Progressively use less and less assistance from the suspension trainer to progress to a bodyweight split squat. You can also use a dowel, a bench, or a band to assist with this movement if a suspension trainer is not available.

GOBLET SPRINTER STEP-UP

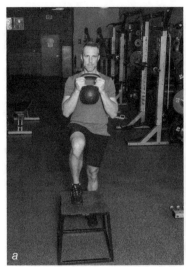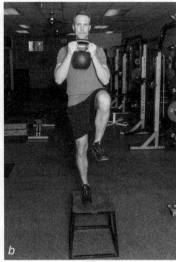

Setup and Performance

- Use a very sturdy box or an adjustable step that will place the thigh approximately parallel to the ground when one foot is placed on top of the step. A 14- to 18-inch (36-46 cm) step tends to be a good height range depending on the height of your client.
- Stand facing the step holding a single dumbbell or kettlebell in the goblet position and place one foot completely on the front part of the step. Keep this foot on the step until all reps have been completed on that leg.
- Pushing primarily through the foot that is on the step, raise yourself up so that you are standing tall on the step on the front leg. The trailing leg will come through without touching the step into a triple flexed (hip, knee, ankle) position as the front leg fully straightens.
- Pause at the top, step back down, repeat and then switch sides.

Key Performance Points

- Keep the pelvis (i.e., "belt-line") level and square to the front during the exercise.
- Finish tall before the trailing leg touches the step.
- Make sure that the foot of the trailing leg is pointing forward at the start of each rep.
- Minimize how much the back leg contributes. How much is too much? If the trailing knee bends excessively, it is probably launching you off at the bottom and the weight should be lowered or (if using bodyweight) the step should be lowered.

SINGLE-LEG SQUAT FROM BOX

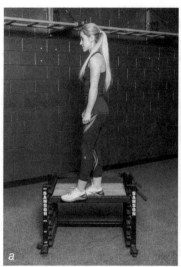 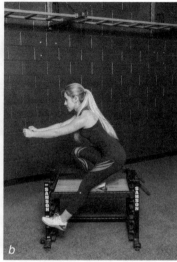

Setup and Performance

- Use a very sturdy box or an adjustable step that will not tip. For most clients, an 18- to 24-inch (46-61 cm) box works well.
- Start on top of the box and stand sideways on the edge of the box with one foot unsupported.
- Reach the arms out in front of the body and squat down and back in a controlled fashion to a position where the top of thigh is below parallel to the ground.

Key Performance Points

- Creating body tension is critical to the success of this movement. Create tension by taking a deep breath, making tight fists, dropping the shoulders away from the ears, and gripping the ground with the standing foot before starting the downward portion of the rep.
- Allow the upper body to fold forward naturally but not excessively, while lowering into the bottom of the squat.

PRISONER BODYWEIGHT ROMANIAN DEADLIFT

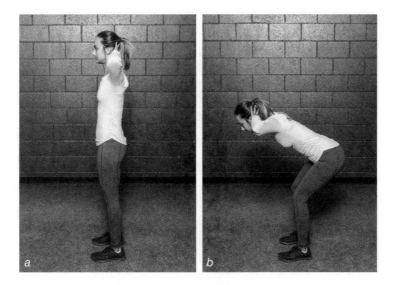

Setup and Performance

- Stand with the feet approximately hip-width apart and the hands placed behind the head with the elbows out.
- Grip the floor with the feet and move the hips backward with a slight knee bend while bending forward. Keep the spine stable while the hips are moving.
- When the hips can not move back any further, return to the starting position and repeat.

Key Performance Points

- We use this drill to teach the proper hip hinge and the concept of moving through the hip joint versus the spine. Keeping the hands behind the head allows for a bit of upper back extension.
- Keep the ribs down and "hidden" slightly to prevent excessive lumbar hyperextension.
- Keep the neck in a relatively neutral position.
- It is often helpful to place the balls of the feet on an elevated block such as a two-by-four or something similar to encourage a posterior weight shift.

DEFICIT DEADLIFT

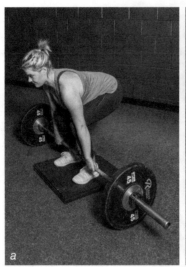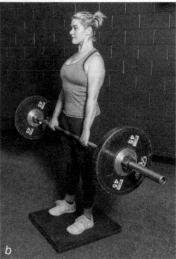

Setup and Performance

- Stand on a solid two- to three-inch (5-8 cm) platform (rubber mats work well).
- The feet will be about hip-width apart or slightly narrower with the bar over the middle of the foot or one to two inches from the shins when standing tall.
- Bend over and grab the bar with an overhand grip or a mixed-grip just outside of the legs.
- Bring the lower legs forward to touch the bar while lifting the chest slightly up to set a rigid and locked position with the armpit right over the middle of the bar. Keep the arms straight.
- Focus on a point about seven to ten feet ahead at the start of the movement.
- Push the floor away and move to a fully standing position, keeping the bar close to the body (lightly touching) from the bottom position to the top.
- Return the bar to the floor by lowering it straight down. The descent should be a mirror image of the ascent. Reset the bar on the floor (i.e. the floor will take the weight of the bar), and repeat.

Key Performance Points

- The deadlift is primarily a hip hinge, not a squat. The biggest mistake that most people make is setting the hips too low at the bottom which actually moves them horizontally further from the barbell. That said, the hips will be a bit lower in this version of the deadlift than they are in a traditional deadlift because standing on the deficit changes some of the relevant angles.
- Create tension and "push" the slack out of the bar *before* attempting to actually lift the bar.

ONE-DUMBBELL SINGLE-LEG ROMANIAN DEADLIFT

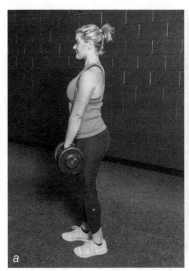 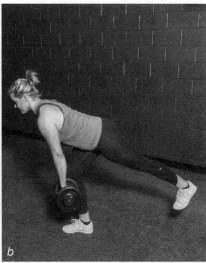

Setup and Performance

- Stand with both feet about hip-width apart and then pick up one foot. The dumbbell should be on the same side as the leg that is going back.
- Hip-hinge on the working leg while the other leg moves back. A straight line should be formed from the rear leg to the head.
- Lower the dumbbell in a straight line to a position that is somewhere between the level of the bottom of the knee and midshin.
- Push the floor away and hip-hinge to return the start position while pulling the dumbbell up in a straight line. Repeat.

Key Performance Points

- In a Romanian deadlift, the exercise starts with the weight at the top of the movement, and the weight will not go the floor or a block to a "dead" weight position.
- Keep the spine stable, and move through the hips. Be sure to establish this position at the beginning, before the lift begins.
- Be sure to keep the working leg bent at the bottom of the movement. This is critical because it allows the hips to move back properly; if the hips don't move back, they will spin open and balance will be compromised.
- Keep the shoulders square at the bottom.

BARBELL SINGLE-LEG ROMANIAN DEADLIFT

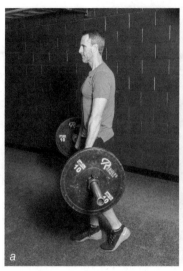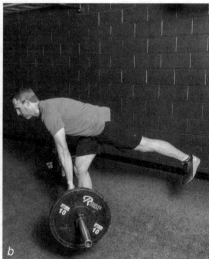

Setup and Performance

- Stand on one foot holding a barbell with a shoulder-width overhand grip and the bar touching the thighs.
- Hip-hinge on one leg, pushing the hip back and bending forward. Lower the barbell down the legs keeping the shoulders square.
- Lower the barbell to just below the bottom of the knees or upper shin depending on individual mobility.
- Push the stance foot into the ground and hip hinge back to the standing position and then repeat.

Key Performance Points

- Keep the back leg extended and relatively low to the ground. A common mistake is to try to lift the leg too high toward the ceiling on the lowering portion of the lift.
- Be sure to keep the stance or working leg bent at the bottom of the movement. This is critical because it allows the hip to move back properly; if the hip doesn't move back, you will rotate open rather than stay squared up to the floor at the bottom of the movement, which will cause balance to be compromised.
- Keep the spine stable and in a relatively straight line during the movement.

SWISS BALL ECCENTRIC-ONLY
SUPINE HIP EXTENSION LEG CURL

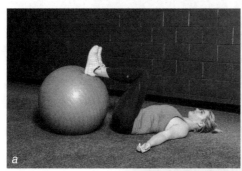
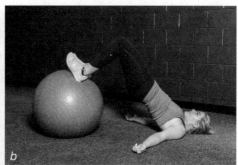
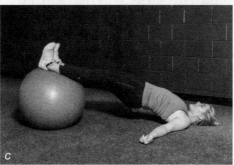

Setup and Performance

- Lie on the floor facing up with the legs straight and the heels together placed on top of a Swiss ball. The arms are at the sides with the palms up.
- Leaving the hips on the floor, pull the Swiss ball toward the butt so the knees are bent.
- Set the core and lift the hips up so that the body forms a straight line from the shoulders, hips, and knees.
- Slowly extend the legs while keeping the hips up and pushing the ball away.
- Maintain the straight line formed between the shoulders, hips, and knees as the ball moves away.

Key Performance Points

- Only the eccentric portion of this exercise is performed, not the concentric.
- Use the arms to stabilize as needed. The position of the arms reduces stability as well.
- Return to the starting point and repeat.

SLIDER SUPINE HIP EXTENSION LEG CURL (SHELC)

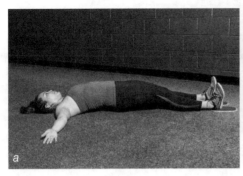
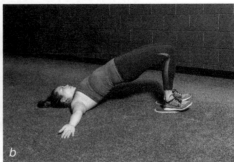

Setup and Performance

- Lie on the floor facing up with the legs straight and the heels together placed on top of a pair of sliders on a sliding surface. The arms are at the sides with the palms up.
- Set the core and lift the hips up so that the body forms a straight line from the shoulders, hips, and knees.
- Pull the heels toward the butt while keeping the hip extended and the core braced. The hips will rise an inch for every inch the heels move back.
- Slowly return to the starting point and repeat.

Key Performance Point

- Bracing the core and maintaining the distance between the ribs and the hips is critical in this movement to prevent excessive lumbar hyperextension.

SUSPENSION TRAINER PUSH-UP

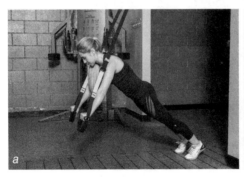
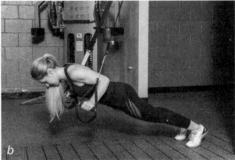

Setup and Performance

- Set the suspension trainer handles in the fully lengthened position.
- Grab the handles and get into a push-up position at a body angle for an appropriately challenging set of repetitions. At the top of the movement the arms will create an approximate 90-degree angle (relative to the torso) as viewed from the side.
- The feet are no wider than hip-width apart.
- Keeping the body in a straight line, lower to the bottom of the push-up and then push back up to the starting position.

Key Performance Points

- Think of this as a moving plank. "Find your plank," on the setup.
- Make sure that the reps are done to the proper depth standard on each rep. The top of the shoulder should be below the elbow at the bottom of the movement.
- At the bottom of the movement the upper arms will be about 45 degrees from the torso when viewed from behind.

T-PUSH-UP

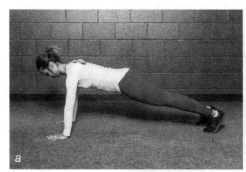 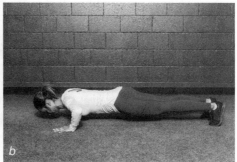

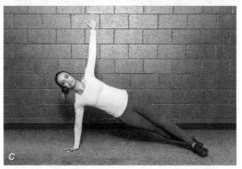

Setup and Performance

- Get into a push-up position with hands very slightly wider than shoulder-width and elbows are straight.
- The feet are slightly wider than hip-width apart.
- In a controlled fashion, lower yourself to the ground keeping the core tight and the upper arms at about a 45-degree angle from the sides.
- As you push up and away from the floor rotate to one side. If the rotation is occurring towards the left, pick up the right hand. Allow the feet to turn simultaneously.
- You will rotate through the shoulders and hips to form a straight line from hand to hand resembling a T shape at the top. Return the hand to the ground, and repeat on the other side.

Key Performance Points

- Be sure the feet have enough room to allow them to pivot to the side.
- The hips and shoulders should move as one unit.
- The T-push is a push-up with a dynamic tall side plank.

DUMBBELL SINGLE-ARM BENCH PRESS

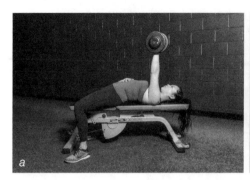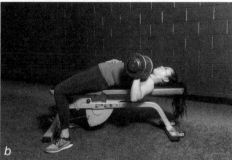

Setup and Performance

- Lie on the back on a flat bench with both feet flat on the floor in a stable position holding one dumbbell directly over the shoulder with the arm straight and vertical.
- Lower the dumbbell to just above the side of the chest and then push back to the starting position.

Key Performance Points

- At the bottom of the movement, the upper arm will be about 45 degrees from the torso.
- Keep the shoulder blades down and back throughout the movement.
- Keep a slight arch in the lower back but keep the butt on the bench.

KETTLEBELL ALTERNATING OVERHEAD PRESS

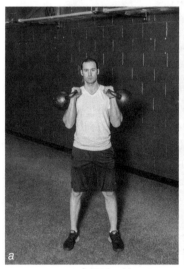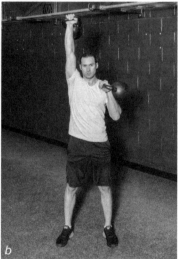

Setup and Performance

- Begin with two kettlebells in the front rack position and the feet about shoulder-width apart. The kettlebells will rest on the wrists and forearms.
- Set the feet approximately shoulder-width apart and "screw" the feet into the floor, tightening the quads, glutes, and grip on both hands.
- Keeping one kettlebell in the rack position, press the other bell up to the top position with the palm facing out. Pull the bell back into the rack position and repeat on the other side.

Key Performance Points

- Keep the wrists neutral and flat.
- Make sure that the pressing arm is straight and vertical at the top as viewed from all angles.
- Keep the legs straight at all times, this is a strict press, not a push press. The knees will be straight but not hyperextended.

CABLE SEATED NEUTRAL-GRIP ROW

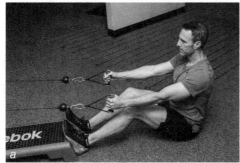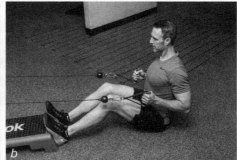

Setup and Performance

- Set the pulley on a functional trainer at approximately knee height in standing, or use a seated cable row machine specifically designed for this exercise.
- Sit on the floor or seat of the unit and grab the handles with the palms facing each other.
- Pull the handles back toward the lower rib cage.
- Return to the starting position and repeat.

Key Performance Points

- Keep the torso relatively vertical throughout the rowing motion.
- Initiate the pull with the shoulder blade rather than the elbow.
- Be sure that the shoulder blades move with the upper arm as opposed to only bending the elbow.

CABLE KNEELING NEUTRAL-GRIP PULLDOWN

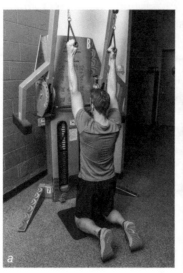 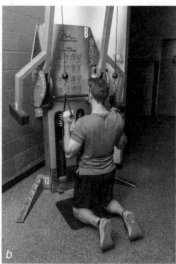

Setup and Performance

- Attach two handles to a high pulley on a functional trainer or a similar configuration.
- Grasp the handles and get into a tall-kneeling posture with the palms facing each other.
- Leading with the shoulder blades, pull down so that the upper arms end at the sides of the torso.
- Return to the starting point and repeat.

Key Performance Points

- Keep the shoulder away from the ears in the bottom position.
- Brace the core and keep the ribs and hips together to maintain the "core cylinder."

ECCENTRIC-ONLY CHIN-UP

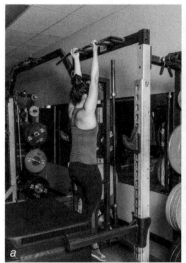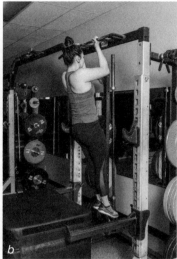

Setup and Performance

- Climb up to the pull-up bar and take about a shoulder-width underhand grip on the bar.
- Get into the top of a chin-up with the chest touching the bar and the arms bent. With control, slowly lower to the bottom position at the assigned cadence.
- Climb back up to the starting position and repeat.

Key Performance Points

- Only the eccentric or lowering phase is performed. It's best to use a tall box if possible to start at the top of the chin-up so that one can simply step off without excessive swinging.
- Brace the core by locking the ribs and hips together before lowering.
- Keep shoulder blades down "in the back pockets" away from the ears.

PART II

The Training Programs

CHAPTER 4

Fat-Loss Programs

One thing that our gym is most renowned for is our approach to attacking fat loss; it's the training topic that we are asked to speak on more than any other. Our society is currently in the middle of an obesity epidemic. In the United States alone, approximately one-third of the adult population is estimated to be obese. In the year 2000, obesity caused 400,000 U.S. deaths, more than 16 percent of all preventable causes of deaths, and the number two killer behind smoking, which accounted for 435,000, or 18 percent, as the number one preventable cause.

Considering these statistics, it might seem that the fitness profession as a whole has failed to make a difference. But it seems that now, at least, people are turning to the fitness industry for help. In the following pages, we are going to take a look at why we need a better approach to fat-loss programs, present some general physiology to understand the principles behind training for fat loss, and then explain its application as we create programs for the goal of fat loss.

The Necessity for Better Fat-Loss Programs

In the past, people were leaner and moved more. The purpose of an exercise program 30 years ago was to enhance an already active lifestyle. Now in an almost completely digital, automated, and time-crunched society, we have had to create exercise programs specifically to induce fat loss. The average person spends more and more time sitting in front a of a TV, smartphone, or computer screen. Despite the overwhelming amount of research on aerobic training and exercise for health in the past, none of it had the primary goal of fat loss in mind.

The fitness industry now recognizes the need to specifically create effective fat-loss programs. We previously didn't know where to start. We originally designed fat-loss programs by copying the programs of endurance athletes, somehow hoping that the training program of a marathon runner would work as a fat-loss program for an obese lady, even when reduced and modified to 20 minutes, three times per week. But fat loss was never the primary goal of an endurance athlete, it was simply a potential side effect.

The fitness industry next turned to bodybuilding for ideas. This was the height of the body-for-life physique transformation contests. And we failed again. To take the programs of full-time professional bodybuilders and use them to model fat-loss programs for the general population was nonsensical. But we tried.

Bodybuilders just happen to be some of the most dedicated and driven people on the planet. I can remember speaking at a seminar with a national-level bodybuilder. He got up two hours before the event so that he could do cardio. He brought all his meals with him in a large Igloo ice chest for the weekend, and he constantly had a gallon of water with him. My point is that it's probably the dedication and discipline that makes a bodybuilder's approach work. So without that dedication, how can we adapt those programs to the average person?

Next, the supplement companies jumped on board to try to convince us that taking brand Rx-O-Plex would provide the same benefits as the drugs that some bodybuilders were using. We failed again, but we were getting closer.

Unlike endurance athletes, fat loss was at least a goal for bodybuilders, but the low percentages of body fat that contest bodybuilders achieved was largely due to their increased muscle mass, and therefore their metabolism. However, it would be naive of us to ignore the impact that steroid use has had on bodybuilding physiques. There is very little information that drug-free, general-population clients, who train three to four times a week, can take from the program of a drug-using, professional body-builder and effectively apply it to their own efforts.

It is our belief that before we start to create a program for fat loss, we have to understand exactly how it occurs. Then we design the program based on those principles and not on tradition, junk science, or outdated beliefs.

Despite advances in the methods of training, the fitness industry has yet to provide a complete fat-loss solution. We have regurgitated programs for other goals, recommended the wrong diets and ineffective exercises plans, and never questioned the origins of this information. This chapter is designed to cut through the junk science and the poor recommendations that the media and, to some degree, the fitness industry have continued to propagate for the last 20 to 30 years. This chapter is a combination of what the scientific literature has taught us regarding fat loss, what we have personally experienced in our facility working with clients, and what our colleagues have found to be effective in their businesses. And it provides a resource of solid principles to design effective fat-loss programs.

The Process of Fat Loss

The bad news is that there is no secret to fat loss. High carbohydrate, low fat? Don't eat fat and you won't get fat? Aerobics to lose fat? "Fat burning" zone? All of these may sound like the secret to fat loss, but none have ever panned out in the real world. We have also explained and detailed the fallacy of focusing on steady-state aerobic training for fat loss in previous works. Suffice it to say that it may be the biggest single lie ever told by the fitness industry. (Okay, maybe the second biggest lie ever. The first, of course, is "the check is in the mail.")

The good news is that fat loss is a simple concept. Simple, yes, but far from easy. It is a simple process that unfortunately requires hard work and a long-term approach. There are no quick fixes. Yes, it requires effort, but to be honest, once you understand fat mobilization and fat metabolism, the process is not too complicated.

Understanding Metabolism and Fat Loss

If you understand how the body burns calories (and therefore burns excess body fat), then you can quickly and easily evaluate most fat-loss programs to see if they fulfill the requirements.

The first part of understanding the fat-loss process is to understand metabolism or metabolic rate. We've all heard phrases such as, "He has a slow metabolism," or "I have a fast metabolism," usually in reference to the difficulty of losing weight or about how much food a person can consume. But what is actually meant by the term *metabolism*?

Put simply, metabolism, or metabolic rate, is the total energy expenditure of the body. Everything that the body does (e.g., breathing, heart rate), requires a certain amount of energy. The rate differs significantly from person to person. You and a friend can have the same activity level, diet, and weight, but still gain or lose weight at different rates based on differences in metabolism.

The process of combining food with oxygen (the burning of calories) releases the energy needed to function. As already stated, every activity that happens in the body requires amount of energy. The total sum of all these actions is measured in calories (essentially a unit of heat), which is known as metabolism or metabolic rate (the rate at which the body consumes energy). The largest percentage of total metabolism (60%-70%) is resting metabolic rate (RMR), sometimes referred to as resting energy expenditure. This is the amount of calories required to maintain the body and its basic functions in a temperate environment while at complete rest—in other words, no activity.

Essentially, metabolism is how many calories a person burns in a typical day and it is affected and controlled by the thyroid and muscle mass. To break it down further, every pound of muscle gained requires the burning of additional calories per day to maintain that muscle. The more muscle a person carries, the higher the resting metabolic rate—hence, an important reason to develop, work, and maintain muscle in any fat-loss program. Hint: This is otherwise known as strength or resistance training.

Additional metabolic demands come from the thermic effect of food (TEF). In a nutshell, the thermic effect of food is a measure of the energy costs required to process certain foods. Some foods require more energy to digest and process than others. Typically, TEF can account for approximately 10 to 20 percent of metabolism. Fat has a very low TEF of approximately three percent of the consumed calories, while protein is a lot higher at approximately 30 percent. We can potentially increase this with careful manipulation of macronutrients and meal frequency.

The balance of a body's caloric needs comes from activity level (another 20%-30%). This is the easiest part to understand and adjust and has become the sole focus of most fat-loss programs. The energy cost of activities such as aerobic training has led us to believe that it is a superior approach to fat loss when compared to anaerobic training such as interval training or resistance training (because less calories are burned during compared to aerobic activity). This is an inherently flawed approach and we'll cover it in more detail later (aerobic work does not necessarily maintain muscle and can actually lower resting metabolic rate). However, when exercise routines are performed correctly, we can create a caloric deficit that will require stored energy to be used (i.e., fat burning).

Increasing Metabolism

Daily energy expenditure consists of three components: Resting metabolic rate (RMR minus the sum of BMR plus basic living), diet-induced thermogenesis (DIT), and energy cost of physical activity (see figure 4.1).

Often, when you explain this to potential fat-loss clients, their first instinct is to decide that they will determine their resting metabolic rate (the amount just needed to survive) and only consume calories for that number, or even below. They think that all their additional metabolic demands (the thermic effect of feeding and activities) will create a massive deficit so that they will lose fat rapidly.

While it's true that the idea of any fat-loss plan is to cut calories and create a gap between intake and

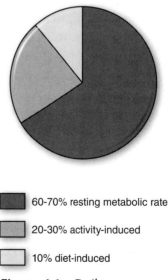

■ 60-70% resting metabolic rate

▨ 20-30% activity-induced

☐ 10% diet-induced

Figure 4.1   Daily energy expenditure.

output, with the goal of burning fat stores, it's important to note that when we consume too few calories to support basic functions, the body simply slows down everything because it doesn't have enough energy to function efficiently.

Extreme low-calorie diets don't necessarily expend more body fat. Instead, muscle is burned (it's easier for the body: four calories per gram for muscle (protein) instead of nine calories per gram for fat). Lean muscle is a major factor in resting metabolic rate, so losing muscle will actually cause metabolism to decrease quickly. Maybe someone used to burn 2,000 calories per day at rest, but after losing a few pounds of muscle, now burns only 1,800 calories or so. Therefore, it becomes very easy to eat less than ever but actually gain weight because there is no longer a deficit. At our facility, we have found that the majority of clients, especially women, have a lifetime history of dieting and have lost muscle, as described previously, over and over again by eating low-calorie diets. Eventually, their bodies get to a point where their muscle mass, and therefore metabolism, is so low that previously effective low-calorie diets no longer work, and they decide to hire a professional. By the time they turn to us they usually have a history of low-calorie diets that we have to undo.

Increasing activity levels and increasing muscle, with the result of increasing RMR is a more effective approach than just cutting calories from the diet. Dieting deprives the body of energy, and that works to an extent, but ramping up the system demands is the more effective way to go. Therefore, a metabolic resistance training program is key; this not only increases calories burned, but it also forces the body to recognize muscle, meaning that during a caloric deficit it will burn fat stores, not muscle. Acknowledging muscle as it pertains to exercise is one of the most important factors in changing body composition (body fat to lean tissue ratio). In other words, exercise designed to grow, or at least maintain, muscle (i.e., resistance exercise) is one of the most important factors in an exercise program designed to change a person's ratio of body fat to total body weight.

In summary, our goal when designing fat-loss programs is to increase metabolic rate to accomplish the following:

- Burn as many calories as possible through resting metabolic rate (lean muscle is metabolically active so building muscle, or at least maintaining it, is extremely important).
- Burn more calories through the thermic effect of food by adjusting meal frequency and manipulating macronutrients. (The thermic effect of protein is twice as high as the thermic effect of fat or carbohydrate.)
- Burn calories through metabolic disturbance (increased activity levels and EPOC).
- Create a gap between total metabolism (calories burned) and intake (calories consumed). In addition, increase calories burned so that calories consumed can be as high as possible. If this situation is met, and adequate protein is consumed and an effective resistance training program is implemented, the body will borrow from its fat stores.

Creating a Fat-Loss Effect

Here is a very simple explanation of what occurs to create a fat-loss effect, or what is commonly referred to as "burning fat." It is a three-step process, which includes mobilization, transport, and oxidation.

Step 1: Mobilization

Subcutaneous fat exists in fat cells. In order to lose fat, we need to transfer it from the cell to the muscle where it can be burned off as energy. This can be accomplished by a caloric deficit. The body needs to recognize a fuel shortage for the required activities so it will draw on some of its energy stores.

The body has three energy stores (nutrients) it can use for fuel:

- Carbohydrate (stored glycogen)
- Protein (lean muscle tissue)
- Fat (stored body fat)

Our basic strategy is to keep the body's glycogen levels low (with diet and intense exercise) so that the body can't draw from its store of carbohydrate. We also want to compel the body to maintain or develop muscle and uphold an anabolic state, or state of positive protein synthesis. Therefore, a reduced carbohydrate diet and a solid weight training program—under conditions of a caloric deficit—will briefly shift the body toward burning fat from its stores.

So how do we remove the fat from those fat cells so that we can actually use it as a fuel source? Mobilizing body fat requires that the triglyceride within the fat cell breaks down into free fatty acids so it can enter the bloodstream. When blood sugar is low, glucagon signals the fat cells to activate hormone sensitive lipase (HSL), and to convert triglycerides into free fatty acids, and transport them to the muscle and liver where they can be burned. This breakdown is limited by HSL levels and is referred to as a *rate-determining step* (RDS).

A rate-determining step is the slowest step in a metabolic pathway or series of chemical reactions, which determines the overall rate of the other reactions in the pathway. In an enzymatic reaction, the rate-limiting step is generally the stage that requires the greatest activation energy or the transition state of highest free energy ("Rate-limiting step").

It's an oversimplification, but if HSL levels are low, then fat mobilization slows down. If we ramp up HSL, fat mobilization will increase. The goal is to increase HSL levels by increasing catecholamine levels in the blood, and we do that through exercise. The higher the intensity the better, because exercise intensity is directly related to increased catecholamine release. Exercising with higher intensity will elevate catecholamine and HSL levels, and therefore increase fat mobilization.

Insulin level is another rate-determining step. The body secretes insulin to remove glucose from the bloodstream. Insulin levels also limit HSL levels, therefore affecting fat mobilization. The basic strategy for mobilizing fat is to maintain low insulin levels and high catecholamine levels. We can lower insulin by keeping blood sugar under control, particularly through exercise and by following a reduced carbohydrate diet. Exercise also elevates catecholamines.

Steps 2 and 3: Transport and Oxidation

If HSL is high, fat cells then break down into free fatty acids (FFA), which are transported in the blood to the muscle where they can be used as fuel. But there's yet another rate-determining step that can slow down or significantly blunt fat loss: carnitine levels. Carnitine levels control the transport of the FFA to the mitochondria, the "powerhouse of the body" where it's actually burned off in the muscle. Basically, the higher the carnitine levels, the higher the rate of fat transport. Increasing carnitine levels will increase mitochondria activity.

Here is a very oversimplified analogy: Think of carnitine as the officials at immigration or passport control, and the process of fat burning equal to leaving the airport. If you were to arrive in a foreign country with 500 other passengers and there was only one official at passport control, it would take a long time to get through immigration and leave the airport. If there were 500 officials, then you would move rapidly through passport control and could leave the airport quickly. The more officials (carnitine) the easier and faster the process of leaving the airport (fat being burned).

To increase carnitine levels we run into another rate-determining step: muscle glycogen levels. (It is interesting that every rate-determining step is limited by a second rate-determining step.) Muscle glycogen levels have to be low for carnitine levels to be high, so in order to have optimal fat oxidation, we need to deplete muscle glycogen through metabolic work (i.e., resistance training or interval training) and dieting (a reduced carbohydrate diet will reduce glycogen levels). When we put that together, we have a simple equation:

high levels of fat mobilization + high levels of fat oxidation = accelerated fat loss

As a side note, waste products released during these reactions are filtered and excreted by the kidneys, but the kidneys need water to do their job effectively. If you are well hydrated, most of your body's waste products can be eliminated through the kidneys. When you are underhydrated, much of this burden is assumed by the liver. As previously mentioned, one of the liver's main functions is processing stored body fat for use as energy. If your kidneys are backed up, the liver helps out (eliminating waste is much more important in the hierarchy of survival than losing fat). The liver will be less efficient at mobilizing body fat if it is busy processing waste products; therefore, proper hydration is also a key to optimal fat loss.

When we develop a strategy to integrate these steps and circumvent each rate-limiting step, we find that fat loss is actually very simple. Again, simple doesn't mean easy but as you can see, we can potentially accelerate fat loss very effectively with the combination one-two punch of reduced carbohydrate intake and intense exercise.

Hierarchy of Fat-Loss Methods

After years of applying various science-based methods to burn the most amount of fat in the least amount of time, we have created what we call the *hierarchy of fat loss* (figure 4.2) (Cosgrove 2007). Based on the previously covered topics, we can construct

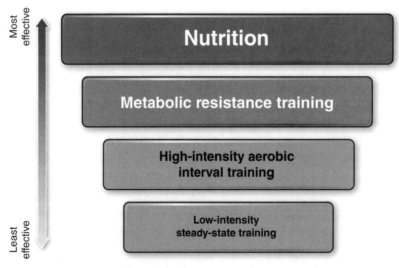

Figure 4.2 Hierarchy of fat loss.

a list of prioritized strategies to attack fat loss, which then helps to prioritize the most effective strategies for our clients based on their available time to train in a given week.

From this, we can rank our priorities for fat-loss training:

1. Metabolic acceleration resistance training and strength training (these are tied)
2. High-intensity anaerobic interval training
3. High-intensity aerobic training
4. Low-intensity aerobic training (steady state)

With these priorities in mind, we can create guidelines based on the client's weekly available training time:

- Three to four available hours per week: use priority 1 exclusively
- Four to five available hours per week: use priorities 1 and 2
- Five to six available hours per week: use priorities 1, 2, and 3
- More than six available hours per week: use priorities 1, 2, 3, and 4

Table 4.1 shows how to apply the hierarchy to a weekly training schedule based on the client's available time. For the sake of illustration, each session is equivalent to an hour.

In our experience at our facility (currently serving approximately 300 clients two to three times per week), in terms of *fat loss*, total body workouts outperform body-part split routines or upper and lower body split routines. That's not to suggest we use the same exercises and movements for every workout, but we try to involve the entire body (training most of the movement patterns) every time we're in the gym. We do use split routines; we just don't assign it based on the muscles involved. (More on this in the next chapter.)

In summary, the only limited and nonrenewable resource is time. Because of this, we must maximize the benefits of a resistance training program by creating maximal

Table 4.1   Example Weekly Sessions Based on Fat-Loss Training Hierarchy and Training Time Available

Session Frequency	Mon	Tues	Wed	Thurs	Fri	Sat	Sun
1-2/week	Resistance training Day A or B			Resistance training Day A or B			
3/week	Resistance training Day A or B		Resistance training Day A or B		Resistance training Day A or B		
4/week	Resistance training Day A or B		Resistance training Day A or B		Resistance training Day A or B	Metabolic interval session	
5/week	Resistance training Day A or B	Metabolic interval session	Resistance training Day A or B		Resistance training Day A or B	Low-intensity or metabolic interval session	

metabolic disturbance, also known as metabolic resistance training. This can be characterized by the following principles:

- *Use heavy resistance relative to repetitions.* This simply means to engage in heavy resistance exercise. Light weight, high reps is a myth. We use near-maximal effort loads, regardless of rep range. Typically, we favor the traditional hypertrophy rep range of 6 to 15 reps, although with more advanced clients we may use an undulating periodization plan, or intermittently add one to two heavier sets (usually in the five to eight rep range) at the beginning of each workout. We use the hypertrophy rep ranges because what builds muscle is what retains muscle; your body needs a reason to hold on to the current muscle and potentially add new lean mass.
- *Time under tensions should approach 45 to 60 seconds.* Load is not the only factor when designing resistance training programs; the actual time exposed to the load is also important. Neural effects (i.e., pure strength) can be maximized by shorter time under tensions (20 seconds or so), while muscular demand can be

Afterburn Effect

In our gym, we call excess post-oxygen consumption (EPOC), the *afterburn effect*. Recent studies have disputed the overall contribution of EPOC to the caloric burn of exercise, suggesting that its involvement is much less than we once thought (although these studies have tended to only focus on aerobic exercise). Sometimes the research disputes the mechanism by which we think something works, but it doesn't dispute what actually works. For example, it is widely accepted that interval training and weight training, despite burning less calories during the session, results in significantly greater fat loss than from longer sessions of lower-intensity activity.

In isocaloric comparisons (i.e., in which the sessions burn the same total amount of calories) weight training always results in greater fat loss than aerobic training. The mechanism by which it works is definitely outside the workout period—an adaptation. We have suggested that it is primarily EPOC or an increase in resting metabolic rate (RMR), but there's recently been discussion on EPOC's actual degree of effect. Other experts have suggested that the increased fat loss could be part EPOC, part elevated fat oxidation, and part increased mitochondrial enzyme activity. So, it may not be an EPOC-related phenomenon only, but it's still a post-workout effect that results in additional fat burning.

Regarding the research dispute: As practitioners, we don't really need to know *why* something works. We are only interested in what actually works and what will repeatedly work with clients. Our suggestion is to focus on the activities that we know to work for fat loss, and let the researchers discover the exact mechanisms behind them.

Essentially, the goal when designing a fat-loss training program is to massively disrupt the metabolism and create as much of a caloric deficit as possible while maximizing the afterburn effect. We increase fat loss by creating a caloric deficit with a reduced carbohydrate diet. We then burn calories through the judicious use of a resistance training program combined with an interval training program. This combination will not only burn a lot of calories during the workout, but it will also crank up the afterburn effect and allow us to continue to burn an elevated amount of fat and calories for several hours after each session.

maximized following a longer time under load. Of course, reps are units of time and it is critical that we are above an effective tension threshold whenever we consider time under tension concepts.

- *Undertake relatively short rest periods by using alternating sets or minicircuits to maximize work density.* The paradox of resistance training for fat loss is how to combine heavy resistance with short rest periods. Usually the two do not go hand in hand! But short rest periods are critical to increasing caloric burn and total work performed. We can assist by using alternating sets to maximize work density. Instead of typical straight set programs, we can work noncompeting body parts (usually alternating upper- and lower-body exercises) in bisets (two exercises), or trisets (three exercises) of circuits to allow us to work harder and with greater resistance, such as this biset pairing example:

  1a: Goblet squats: 2 to 3 sets of 8 to 12 reps with 60-second rest

  1b: Dumbbell bench rows: 2 to 3 sets of 8 to 12 reps with 60-second rest

If each set takes almost one minute to complete, the lower body and upper body each get approximately three minutes of rest between sets. This allows the use of very heavy weights, because a three-minute rest period for the muscle group is more than enough to allow for recovery in the 8 to 12 rep range. However, actual rest time is only 60 seconds. By pairing upper and lower body in an alternating fashion we can drastically increase total work done in the same time period, therefore increasing total calories burned and significantly increasing EPOC.

With all of these factors in mind, the fastest way to achieve desired results for the typical time-crunched person is

- two to three resistance training sessions per week, and
- one to two metabolic interval sessions per week.

Combined with a reduced refined-carbohydrate diet and targeted supplementation and food selection, this plan can easily result in one to three pounds of fat loss per week.

Fat-Loss Programming

Let's get into the nitty-gritty and introduce two phases of our resistance training programming for fat-loss clients. We will first share two phases of a beginner/intermediate program and then two phases of a more advanced program.

Beginner to Intermediate Program

This program is designed to be used primarily by clients who scored below 15 on our training age rubric discussed in chapter 2. That said, it is still effective for those that scored over 15, so anyone with the goal of fat loss can start with this resistance training program.

The client will alternate between session A and session B on each training day, performing session A six times and session B six times in each phase. Phases 1 and 2 are each designed to be done for four to six weeks depending on how frequently the client trains each week. This also provides some flexibility. If the client trains with a frequency of three times per week (see table 4.2), phase 1 and 2 will each be completed in four weeks, and if training two times per week (see table 4.3), it will take six weeks to complete each phase. After completing all of the A and B sessions for phase 1, the client moves on to phase 2. See tables 4.4 through 4.7 for the sample beginner to intermediate fat-loss program.

Interval Work

We have prescribed interval training in the energy system component in these fat-loss phases, for both the beginner/intermediate and advanced programs. This is an optional piece depending on the conditioning level of the client going into phase 1. Intervals may not be the best choice if your client is reluctant or if time is a limiting factor. In this case, focus on resistance training and preparing the muscular system because this is the priority and it will have the highest return on investment.

It's important to note that we schedule intervals at the end of resistance training sessions for clients who are not doing separate high-intensity interval sessions on separate days as separate sessions. If clients are performing high-intensity intervals on nonresistance training days, we will typically not schedule intervals at the end of their resistance training sessions because the training dosage will become excessive.

Here is an example of how to perform the intervals: If we prescribe 5 to 10 sets of 15 second "hard" and 45 second "easy" intervals, this equates to 5 to 10 total minutes of work. It is listed as a range so that one set (or round) can be added each week. It should also be stated that "hard" means getting after it and really putting forth effort. This directive often needs to be precisely explained by a coach to be fully understood. In our gym we have the luxury of having various equipment options available to perform these intervals. We like to choose modalities that allow for a high relative power output and tend to have a lower technical demand. Here are a few examples for interval work:

Fan bike
Various medicine ball throws
Battling ropes
Sled push and drag
Stair stepper
Climbing machine
Rowing machine
Sprint on a nonmotorized treadmill
Kettlebell swing (if client is qualified)

You can pick one modality and use that for the day, or mix and match using different exercises (choosing up to four different exercises and alternating between them on each set). There are several other applicable exercises in the "Shred" team training programs in chapter 8.

Table 4.2 Beginner to Intermediate Phase 1 and 2 Sample Weekly Schedule: Three Sessions per Week

	Mon	Tues	Wed	Thurs	Fri	Sat	Sun
Week 1	Session A		Session B		Session A		
Week 2	Session B		Session A		Session B		
Week 3	Session A		Session B		Session A		
Week 4	Session B		Session A		Session B		

Table 4.3   Beginner to Intermediate Phase 1 and 2 Sample Weekly Schedule: Two Sessions per Week

	Mon	Tues	Wed	Thurs	Fri	Sat	Sun
Week 1	Session A			Session B			
Week 2	Session A			Session B			
Week 3	Session A			Session B			
Week 4	Session A			Session B			
Week 5	Session A			Session B			
Week 6	Session A			Session B			

Table 4.4   Beginner to Intermediate Fat-Loss Program: Phase 1, Day A

Core training			SETS	REPS	TEMPO	REST
	1a.	Front plank	1-2	1	30-45 sec	0 sec
	1b.	Cable tall-kneeling antirotation press	1-2	10 each side	1-3-1	60 sec
Resistance training			SETS	REPS	TEMPO	REST
	2a.	Goblet squat	1-3	12-15	—	60 sec
	2b.	Cable half-kneeling single-arm row	1-3	12-15 each side	Mod	60 sec*
	3a.	One-dumbbell staggered-stance Romanian deadlift	1-3	12 each side	—	60 sec
	3b.	Push-up	1-3	12	—	60 sec*
Energy systems training			SETS	WORK	RECOVERY	
	4.	Interval	5-10	15 sec	45 sec	

*During this rest period, clients will often perform a mobility and stability drill based on their FMS results and tailored to their needs, so it may be something like an active hip flexor stretch, a "rib pull" (thoracic spine rotation drill), or an ankle mobility drill.

Table 4.5   Beginner to Intermediate Fat-Loss Program: Phase 1, Day B

Core training			SETS	REPS	TEMPO	REST
	1a.	Sandbag dead bug with alternating leg reach	1-2	5 each side	FE	0 sec
	1b.	Side plank from knees	1-2	4-6 each side	5 sec	60 sec
Resistance training			SETS	REPS	TEMPO	REST
	2a.	Kettlebell deadlift	1-3	12-15	—	60 sec
	2b.	Kettlebell half-kneeling single-arm overhead press	1-3	12-15 each side	—	60 sec*
	3a.	Goblet split squat	1-3	12 each side	—	60 sec
	3b.	Kneeling neutral-grip pulldowns	1-3	12-15	—	60 sec*
Energy systems training			SETS	WORK	RECOVERY	
	4.	Interval	5-10	15 sec	45 sec	

*During this rest period, clients will often perform a mobility and stability drill based on their FMS results and tailored to their needs, so it may be something like an active hip flexor stretch, a "rib pull" (thoracic spine rotation drill), or an ankle mobility drill.

Table 4.6   Beginner to Intermediate Fat-Loss Program: Phase 2, Day A

Core training			SETS	REPS	TEMPO	REST
	1a.	Suspension trainer front plank	1-2	1	30-45 sec	0 sec
	1b.	Cable bar half-kneeling chops	1-2	8 each side	—	60 sec
Resistance training			SETS	REPS	TEMPO	REST
	2a.	Goblet squat	2-3	8-10	—	60 sec
	2b.	Dumbbell three-point neutral-grip row	2-3	8-10 each side	—	60 sec*
	3a.	One-dumbbell single-leg block deadlift	2-3	10 each side	—	60 sec
	3b.	Feet-elevated or resisted push-up	2-3	8-10	—	60 sec*
Energy systems training			SETS	WORK	RECOVERY	
	4.	Interval	5-10	20 sec	40 sec	

*During this rest period, clients will often perform a mobility and stability drill based on their FMS results and tailored to their needs, so it may be something like an active hip flexor stretch, a "rib pull" (thoracic spine rotation drill), or an ankle mobility drill.

Table 4.7   Beginner to Intermediate Fat-Loss Program: Phase 2, Day B

Core training			SETS	REPS	TEMPO	REST
	1a.	Sandbag full dead bug with alternating leg reach	1-2	5 each side	FE	0 sec
	1b.	Side plank	1-2	4-6 each side	5 sec	60 sec
Resistance training			SETS	REPS	TEMPO	REST
	2a.	High hex bar deadlift	2-3	10	—	60 sec
	2b.	Kettlebell single-arm over-head press	2-3	8-10 each side	—	60 sec*
	3a.	Two-dumbbell split squat	2-3	10 each side	—	60 sec
	3b.	Suspension trainer inverted neutral-grip row	2-3	8-10	Mod	60 sec*
Energy systems training			SETS	WORK	RECOVERY	
	4.	Interval	5-10	20 sec	40 sec	

*During this rest period, clients will often perform a mobility and stability drill based on their FMS results and tailored to their needs, so it may be something like an active hip flexor stretch, a "rib pull" (thoracic spine rotation drill), or an ankle mobility drill.

Advanced Program

This program is designed to be used by clients with a primary goal of fat loss who scored 15 points or above on our training age rubric discussed in chapter 2. It should not be used by clients who scored less than 15 points.

The client will alternate between session A and session B on each training day performing session A six times and session B six times in each phase. Phases 1 and 2 are each designed to be done for four to six weeks depending on how frequently the client trains each week. This also provides some flexibility. If the client trains with a frequency of three times per week (see table 4.8), phases 1 and 2 will each be completed in four weeks, and if training two times per week (see table 4.9), it will take six weeks to complete each phase. After completing all of the A and B sessions for phase 1, the client moves on to phase 2. See tables 4.10 through 4.13 for the sample advanced fat-loss program.

Table 4.8 Advanced Phase 1 and 2 Sample Weekly Schedule: Three Sessions per Week

	Mon	Tues	Wed	Thurs	Fri	Sat	Sun
Week 1	Session A		Session B		Session A		
Week 2	Session B		Session A		Session B		
Week 3	Session A		Session B		Session A		
Week 4	Session B		Session A		Session B		

Table 4.9 Advanced Phase 1 and 2 Sample Weekly Schedule: Two Sessions per Week

	Mon	Tues	Wed	Thurs	Fri	Sat	Sun
Week 1	Session A			Session B			
Week 2	Session A			Session B			
Week 3	Session A			Session B			
Week 4	Session A			Session B			
Week 5	Session A			Session B			
Week 6	Session A			Session B			

Table 4.10 Advanced Fat-Loss Program: Phase 1, Day A

Core training			SETS	REPS	TEMPO	REST
	1a.	Suspension trainer body saw	2	4 each side	3 sec	0 sec
	1b.	Side plank + Cable single-arm row	2	8-10	Slow	60 sec
Resistance training			SETS	REPS	TEMPO	REST
	2a.	Two-kettlebell front squat or Front squat				
		Sessions 1, 2, & 3	2-3	15	—	60 sec
		Sessions 4, 5, & 6	3	12	—	60 sec
	2b.	Dumbbell three-point neutral-grip row				
		Sessions 1, 2, & 3	2-3	15 each side	—	60 sec*
		Sessions 4, 5, & 6	3	12 each side	Mod	60 sec*
	3a.	Swiss ball supine hip extension leg curl (SHELC)				
		Sessions 1, 2, & 3	2-3	15	2-1-2	60 sec
		Sessions 4, 5, & 6	3	12	3-2-3	60 sec
	3b.	Single-leg push-up (alternate leg each set)				
		Sessions 1, 2, & 3	2-3	15	—	60 sec*
		Sessions 4, 5, & 6	3	12	—	60 sec*
Energy systems training			SETS	WORK	RECOVERY	
	4.	Interval	4-7	30 sec	60 sec	

*During this rest period, clients will often perform a mobility and stability drill tailored to their needs and based on their FMS results, so it may be something like an active hip flexor stretch, a "rib pull" (thoracic spine rotation drill), or an ankle mobility drill.

Table 4.11 Advanced Fat-Loss Program: Phase 1, Day B

Core training			SETS	REPS	TEMPO	REST
	1a.	Sandbag tall-plank lateral isometric hold	2	4 each side	3 sec	0 sec
	1b.	Suspension trainer prone jackknife	2	8-10	Slow	60 sec
Resistance training			SETS	REPS	TEMPO	REST
	2a.	High hex bar deadlift				
		Sessions 1, 2, & 3	2-3	15	—	60 sec
		Sessions 4, 5, & 6	3	12	—	60 sec
	2b.	Two-dumbbell overhead Arnold press				
		Sessions 1, 2, & 3	2-3	12-15	Mod	60 sec*
		Sessions 4, 5, & 6	3	10-12	Mod	60 sec*
	3a.	Goblet rear-foot elevated split squat				
		Sessions 1, 2, & 3	2-3	15 each side	—	60 sec
		Sessions 4, 5, & 6	3	12 each side	—	60 sec
	3b.	Suspension trainer inverted neutral-grip rows				
		Sessions 1, 2, & 3	2-3	15	Mod	60 sec*
		Sessions 4, 5, & 6	3	12	Mod	60 sec*
Energy systems training			SETS	WORK	RECOVERY	
	4.	Interval	3-6	30 sec	60 sec	

*During this rest period, clients will often perform a mobility and stability drill tailored to their needs and based on their FMS, so it may be something like an active hip flexor stretch, a "rib pull" (thoracic spine rotation drill), or an ankle mobility drill.

Table 4.12 Advanced Fat-Loss Program: Phase 2, Day A

Core training			SETS	REPS	TEMPO	REST
	1a.	Suspension trainer prone plank	2	6-8	Slow	0 sec
	1b.	Sandbag tall-plank lateral drag	2	5 each side	Slow	60 sec
Resistance training			SETS	REPS	TEMPO	REST
	2a.	Deadlift	2-3	10	—	0 sec (or as little as necessary)
	2b.	Barbell overhead press	2-3	10	—	0 sec
	2c.	Single-leg skater squat	2-3	10 each side	—	120 sec
	3a.	One-dumbbell hand-supported single-leg neutral-grip row	2-3	10 each side	—	0 sec
	3b.	Suspension trainer push-up + prone jackknife	2-3	8-10	—	90 sec
Energy systems training			SETS	WORK	RECOVERY	
	4.	Interval	6-10	30 sec	30 sec	

*During this rest period, clients will often perform a mobility and stability drill tailored to their needs and based on their FMS results, so it may be something like an active hip flexor stretch, a "rib pull" (thoracic spine rotation drill), or an ankle mobility drill.

Table 4.13   Advanced Fat-Loss Program: Phase 2, Day B

Core training			SETS	REPS	TEMPO	REST
	1a.	Swiss ball fallouts	2	6-10	1-2-1	0 sec
	1b.	Kettlebell single-arm farmer's walk	2	20 yd each side	—	60 sec
Resistance training			**SETS**	**REPS**	**TEMPO**	**REST**
	2a.	Front squat	2-3	10	—	0 sec (or little as necessary)
	2b.	Chin-ups	2-3	5-10	—	0 sec
	2c.	One-dumbbell single-leg Romanian deadlift	2-3	10 each side	—	120 sec
	3a.	Suspension trainer push-up	2-3	10	—	0 sec
	3b.	Low-cable single-arm rotational row	2-3	10 each side	—	90 sec
Energy systems training			**SETS**	**WORK**	**RECOVERY**	
	4.	Interval	6-10	30 sec	30 sec	

*During this rest period, clients will often perform a mobility and stability drill tailored to their needs and based on their FMS results, so it may be something like an active hip flexor stretch, a "rib pull" (thoracic spine rotation drill), or an ankle mobility drill.

ONE-DUMBBELL STAGGERED-STANCE ROMANIAN DEADLIFT

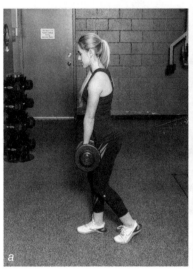 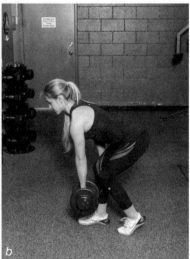

Setup and Performance

- Stand with the feet hip-width apart and slide one foot back so the toe of the back foot is in line with the heel of the front foot or up to a few inches behind it.
- Keep the back heel elevated off the floor, with most of your weight in the front foot. (The back foot serves primarily as a kickstand.)
- Hold one dumbbell in the hand of the back leg opposite, or contra, the front or working leg.
- With soft knees, push the hips back and bend forward, loading the hips.
- Push through the floor with the front foot and return to the starting position.

Key Performance Points

- Keep the spine stable. The movement comes through the hips, not the spine.
- Slide the shoulder blades down toward the back pockets and keep the shoulders square as the hip-hinging occurs.
- A posterior weight shift needs to occur to execute the movement properly; be sure the movement is coming from the hips and not from dropping the chest or arm down. The front shin should stay relatively vertical as if it is in a ski boot.
- Make sure the hips stay level without moving noticeably to the left or right. Keep the hips in the "center lane" as they go back.

CABLE BAR HALF-KNEELING CHOP

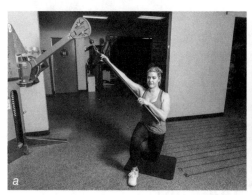 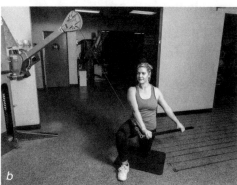

Setup and Performance

- Attach a cable bar or long rope to an adjustable cable machine with a high pulley that is set to approximately head height when standing.
- Get into a half-kneeling position next to the machine and turn perpendicular to the pulley. The inside knee (leg closest to the weight stack) should be up.
- Use an overhand grip and pull the bar across the body, keeping the bar close to the torso, and then move both arms out at the bottom, moving the cable in a diagonal line.

Key Performance Points

- Be sure to keep the torso stacked through the whole movement. Keep the rib cage stacked over the hips. Think of this as a half-kneeling plank.
- There will be some rotation and motion through the upper back and shoulders, but keep the hips static.

SUSPENSION TRAINER INVERTED NEUTRAL-GRIP ROW

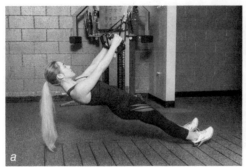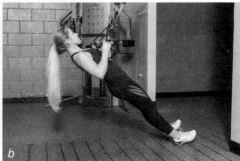

Setup and Performance

- Set the suspension trainer to the short setting so that it is at about hip height.
- Keeping the arms straight and holding onto the handles, walk your feet down to create the proper body angle for an appropriately challenging set of repetitions.
- Holding onto the straps with palms facing each other, keep the heels planted into the ground with toes pulled forward, and find a strong plank position.
- Perform a row by pulling the body toward the anchor point. Note that this is one of the few rowing variations where the hips are extended during the rowing motion.
- Lower yourself back down, maintaining plank position and repeat.

Key Performance Points

- Keep the eyes focused on the anchor point (where the suspension trainer is attached) to help maintain a neutral head and neck position throughout the movement.
- Keep some daylight between the upper arm and torso because this allows the scapula and humerus to work with proper scapulo-thoracic and scapulo-humeral rhythm.
- Spread the chest during the row, or "spread your shirt logo" to properly retract the shoulder blades.
- Be sure that the shoulder blades move with the upper arms, as opposed to only bending the elbows.

SELECT ADVANCED FAT-LOSS PROGRAM EXERCISES

SUSPENSION TRAINER PRONE JACKKNIFE

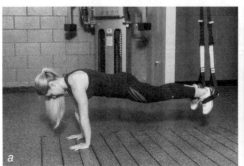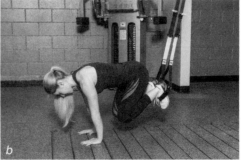

Setup and Performance

- Adjust the bottom of the foot straps so that they hang at midshin.
- Place the foot straps on feet and get into a tall plank position with hands under the shoulders and the feet positioned under the anchor point.
- Bend the knees and hips and bring them towards the arms while keeping the spine stable.
- Return to the starting position and repeat.

Key Performance Points

- Keep the arms straight and keep the wrists stacked under the shoulders.
- Keep the hips and shoulders relatively level while flexing the hip and knees.
- Keep the neck in neutral position; do not "chicken neck."

TWO-DUMBBELL OVERHEAD ARNOLD PRESS

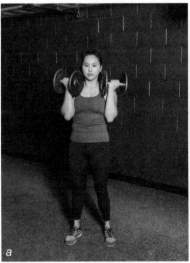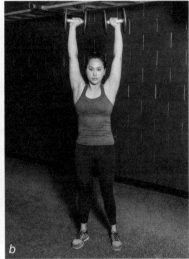

Setup and Performance

- Stand with the feet shoulder-width apart and a dumbbell in each hand in front of the chest, palms facing the body, the arm close to the sides.
- Press the dumbbells toward the ceiling rotating hands from a palm facing-in position to a palm facing-out position.
- Bring the dumbbells back to the starting position, reset, and repeat.

Key Performance Points

- Think about driving the body away from the dumbbells during the pressing motion.
- Imagine you are gripping the floor with the feet to help create full-body tension through this movement.
- "Hide the ribs" to set the proper core position and to keep the core cannister intact while pressing.

LOW-CABLE SINGLE-ARM ROTATIONAL ROW

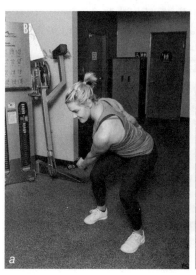 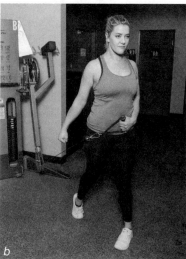

Setup and Performance

- Attach a handle to the low pulley of the machine.
- Stand sideways to the pulley with your feet a bit wider than shoulder-width apart and hips pushed back holding the handle with the outside hand, across your body.
- Sit back and slightly down while turning the shoulders perpendicular to the hips.
- Strongly drive the floor away as you rotate open and pull the handle across your body toward the bottom of the rib cage to finish.
- Return to the starting position, reset, and repeat.

Key Performance Points

- The rotation occurs in the upper back and the hips, not the lumbar spine.
- Be sure to turn the shoulders perpendicular to the hips in the starting position.
- Don't try to hold a long static pause in the end position.

ONE-DUMBBELL HAND-SUPPORTED SINGLE-LEG NEUTRAL-GRIP ROW

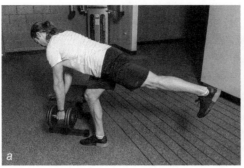 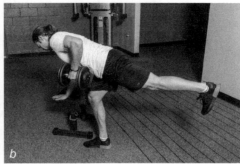

Setup and Performance

- Stand next to a 16- to 18-inch (41-46 cm) bench or box (higher if needed). Hinge over on the inside leg (the leg next to the bench) holding a dumbbell in the hand opposite (or contra) the standing leg.
- The back leg should be extended and straight and the body should almost form a T position. Place the free hand on the bench to provide support and keep the arm straight.
- Pull the dumbbell back toward the bottom of the ribs and slightly outside the body.
- Return to the starting position and repeat.

Key Performance Points

- When rowing, ensure that the shoulder blade is moving. A common error is to only bend the elbow without much, if any, shoulder blade movement. A good cue for all rowing-type movement is to "spread the logo on the front of your t-shirt."
- Bring the dumbbell toward the bottom of the rib cage, not into the armpit.
- Keep the spine relatively straight and stable.

CHAPTER 5

Muscle-Building Programs

Muscle growth, or hypertrophy in exercise physiology terms, is a fairly straightforward process. You stress and challenge the body by lifting heavy objects multiple times, then recover (i.e., eat and provide your body with the proper resources), and your body adapts by getting bigger and stronger. Noted hypertrophy researcher Dr. Brad Schoenfeld (2010, 2011) has proposed that hypertrophy is produced by three primary mechanisms:

- *Mechanical tension*: heavy weight
- *Metabolic stress*: lifting higher reps to failure or getting a "pump"
- *Muscle damage*: microscopic tears in muscle fibers

Of course, the actual physiology of this process goes much deeper. In this chapter, we do not deep-dive into the physiology of muscle hypertrophy. There are a plethora of resources available on muscle hypertrophy, such as Dr. Duncan French's chapter 5, "Adaptations to Anaerobic Training Programs," in the fourth edition of the *NSCA Essentials of Strength Training and Conditioning* (French 2016). In this chapter, we focus on the practical reasons why and how to program for gaining muscle in a general population client.

Should We Emulate Competitive Bodybuilders?

Where many coaches and trainers have typically gone wrong is that they tend to emulate the body-part split training of competitive bodybuilders to accomplish the goal of muscle growth. It is an understandable choice since competitive bodybuilding is all about the pursuit of growing bigger muscles, and these bodybuilders are obviously quite successful. The first problem with this thought process is that most of our clients aren't actually competitive bodybuilders.

The fitness industry has been heavily influenced by bodybuilding since about the 1960s and this influence is still quite strong almost 60 years later as you can see with a quick glance around any commercial gym. We get it. The coaches and clients that are 40 years old or older were subject to a very heavy mainstream bodybuilding influence because the primary sources of information were muscle magazines and the lifters at mainstream gyms. Admittedly, the strong influence of CrossFit has done a lot to change the landscape over the past decade.

Many may think that we are being overly critical of competitive bodybuilding. We would like to make it clear that we appreciate the sport of bodybuilding and we respect competitive bodybuilders. They happen to be some of the most disciplined people on the planet and we want to take nothing away from what they accomplish. There are many things that we have learned and continue to learn from the sport of bodybuilding. We study what successful bodybuilders do, and we apply some of it to our programming. Many things (but not everything) have a time and a place.

Movement Pattern Split Routines for Muscle Building

Over the years, we have often caught some flack for our opposition to body-part or muscle-group split routines. Fundamentally, this is our biggest criticism when it comes to dissecting the actual training of competitive bodybuilders. Body-part allocation to organize your training is purely random and isn't based on any rational physiology. We take issue with how the training is organized, not with bodybuilding itself (we promise that it is nothing personal). Specifically, the problem is not the split routine per se, it is that (1) we need to use some kind of movement-based physiology instead of geography to create the split, and (2) the people who are often doing these splits have no business doing them.

Problem Number 1: Need for Movement-Based Programming

Here is a common muscle group-type split that was posted on an Internet forum several years ago:

Day 1: chest and abs

Day 2: back and biceps

Day 3: rest/cardio/etc.

Day 4: legs and lower back

Day 5: shoulders and triceps

Day 6 and 7: rest/cardio/etc.

Alwyn responded, "Why do shoulders and triceps get the same emphasis as lower back and the entire lower body? Why do triceps get hit twice a week (triceps are included in pushing exercises on Day 1) but abs and biceps only once?" Think about it like this: A bench press uses the chest, shoulders, and triceps. If you have a chest day do you bench press on that day, or save it for the triceps day? What if your triceps are the weakest in the lift and limit what you can do? Does that mean it's not a good chest exercise anymore? Why is the chest more important than the traps? The chest can get its own day, but do traps (they are actually bigger muscles than the pecs, by the way) not deserve their own day too? Or are the traps simply included on back day? We could go on and on, but we will spare you.

We maintain that allocating body parts to separate days isn't based on anything other than choice or preference. It's not science. You can give us examples of bombing and blitzing the biceps and triceps, or trashing the quads all you want, but it doesn't change that simple fact.

There is a lack of logic to using body-part splits; therefore, we prefer not to use them at all and instead organize our training splits based on the movement patterns we displayed earlier in chapter 3. Over the years some critics have confused our stance and have thought that we were against *all* splitting of routines. This is not true. We are not opposed to split routines, but we are not big fans of *body-part* splits. We like to organize training based on what the body does versus where a muscle happens to be.

Interestingly, when we look back at the bodybuilders of yesteryear (prior to the '60s), they tended to train the body as a unit and did not treat it as a collection of individual parts, as though it were Frankenstein's monster. These old school bodybuilders appeared to use a body-part *emphasis* to improve lagging body parts in addition to their regular routine (e.g., upper-lower, full-body, or exercise-based). The reality is that the body is an integrated unit and should be trained as an interconnected system. We once again refer the interested reader to Thomas Myers' book *Anatomy Trains* (2001) to show the connections via the various sling systems of the body.

Just as with fat-loss goals discussed in the previous chapter, for the majority of our clients who want to increase muscle mass, we tend to favor an A and B session full-body split, typically with different exercises for the movement patterns on each training day. But remember, the bulk of our hypertrophy clients are regular people looking to get a little more "jacked," not competitive bodybuilders looking to get on stage. When a client advances from the beginner to intermediate phase to the advanced phase, we will sometimes modify their program to an upper and lower split if they are able to train at least three to four days per week. We determine the split based on the client's:

- current training age and status, and
- available training time.

The majority of our athletes (an athlete is anyone looking for strength and performance) also need to work on full-body routines or sometimes upper and lower splits. The topic of strength will be discussed further in chapter 6. We typically use a split in this way for most of the training goals that we pursue in this book.

Many argue that most of this body-part split talk is just semantics, and they may be correct to a degree, but we feel that we have made a strong case as to how splitting up workouts by body part can lead to problems. The lack of rationale behind it leaves the door wide open for errors to be made. If you are going to spend time analyzing which exercises, sets, reps, and rest periods are the most effective based on science, then you have to create a better system of allocating these exercises, sets, and reps rather than by muscle groups.

Problem Number 2: Time Limitations for the Average Person

The second problem with trying to follow a body-part split routine similar to that of a top-level bodybuilder is that for the average person interested in building muscle, time is a major limiting factor. It's just not realistic for the average person to get the necessary work done for a body-part split routine with a limited amount of training time. Remember, in reality, most people have two to three days per week to dedicate to training. Right off the bat you can see how the body-part split stops making sense. It's also not as productive due to the lack of frequency that a body part or muscle group gets trained per week. Full-body routines are the solution to these constraints.

It's prudent to consider the scientific studies that compare training a muscle group once per week versus training it multiple times per week. One study (McLester, Bishop, and Guilliams 2000) compared the same volume of training per muscle per week (e.g., three sets performed once per week [typical of a body-part split routine] versus one set performed three times per week). The one-day-per-week group only achieved 62 percent of the strength improvements of the three-days-per-week group and achieved a lesser increase in muscle. This would be the primary problem with applying the muscle-group allocation to the average client—frequency, and therefore weekly training volume would greatly suffer. Additionally, another review paper (Wernbom et al. 2007) also concluded that training two to three days per week per muscle group was optimal for hypertrophy. Thus, a more frequent approach (appearing to be about two to three times per week) to training each muscle group or a movement pattern appears to be a better choice. If you used a traditional body-part split for clients who could only train two days per week, they would only be able to train some of the muscle groups only one time per week, which is inferior based on the available literature (Schoenfeld et al., "Effects of Low- Versus High-Load Resistance Training," 2015, Schoenfeld et al., "Effects of Resistance Training Frequency on Measures of Muscle Hypertrophy," 2016) and our extensive practical experience.

This, then, begs the question as to whether a body-part split is actually the better option for a competitive bodybuilder. Maybe, or maybe not. We'll concede that a body-part split *may* be better for advanced, competitive bodybuilders, but we don't see much logic to the body-part allocation for *most* people.

That said, basing splits on a movement-pattern split or an upper or lower split still isn't perfect because there are flaws with this classification method too (e.g., if you perform a heavy barbell dead row on "upper" day, it still strongly involves the "lower" hamstrings and glutes). However, it does avoid most of the problems associated with using muscle groups as the basis of organization of training. It currently seems to be the better way, but who knows where we will go next. At the very least, this type of classification is based on functions (joint actions, movements) and it has been a great way to minimize our clients' training-induced injuries and to perform the required training frequency.

Key Variables in Hypertrophy Programming

While all programs contain the primary training variables previously introduced in chapter 1, there are a few specific key variables that are related to the expansive topic of volume and how these variables pertain to hypertrophy. In very simple terms, volume is a descriptor of the amount of work performed. The first three primary training variables discussed in chapter 2 (reps, sets, loading) are all related to training volume or work (as is weekly training frequency, which we'll discuss later). These parameters are interrelated and any one of them discussed without consideration of the others can lead to assumptions, misinterpretations, and misunderstandings.

The number of repetitions will affect all of the other variables and is the most important variable to manipulate as you learn to write programs. The number of reps per set that your program contains will determine how many sets the client will do, how much rest will be prescribed, how much load will be lifted, and the speed at which to lift it. We consider the number of repetitions performed to be the most important acute exercise variable because it can often determine the training effect (motor control, stability, hypertrophy, and maximum strength) and it can influence all other loading parameters: sets, tempo, rest periods, and even exercise selection. If we decide to perform high rep sets, then certain exercises are no longer appropriate selections, and vice versa. Reps are basically the bricks with which we build the house.

When we break down a resistance training session, we can subdivide it into a series of exercises. Beyond the different exercises, all we have is a series of sets. When we break down the sets, all that is left is a series of repetitions. A repetition is merely moving a load from point A to point B at a prescribed rate of movement. Therefore, a rep is a measure of time and distance and can be thought of as one full cycle of the muscle actions involved. Basically, regardless of the training modality used, programming boils down to the prescription of reps. It is also important to recognize that there is often an inverse relationship between sets and reps. As reps increase, sets decrease, and vice versa.

Volume can be a very nebulous word and any training discussion about it needs to start with the question: "What do you mean by volume?" Volume is a major factor when balancing a program to prevent injury, and it has a direct effect on both hypertrophy and strength development. The reason we don't list it in our key variables is because the first three variables (reps, sets, and loading) actually comprise volume, so it is directly addressed by these variables even if it is not specifically listed.

There are three primary ways to define training volume and they all have various problems associated with them because each requires context to give them any meaning.

$$\text{sets} \times \text{reps} \times \text{load} = \text{tonnage or total volume load}$$

$$\text{(e.g., 3 sets} \times 10 \text{ reps} \times 100 \text{ lb} = 3000 \text{ lb total volume load)}$$

$$\text{sets} \times \text{reps} = \text{total number of reps}$$

$$\text{(e.g., 3 sets} \times 10 \text{ reps} = 30 \text{ total reps)}$$

$$\text{total set volume} = \text{number of "hard" sets}$$

$$\text{(e.g., 3 sets} \times 10 \text{ reps} = 3 \text{ hard sets or work sets)}$$

In the first equation, tonnage needs to have a minimum-intensity threshold to have any real relevance, and it is only relevant when comparing lifters' performances to themselves. In the second equation, the total number of repetitions also needs to have a qualifying of intensity, or a threshold of loading and effort, to have much significance. And in the third equation, total set volume is another way of qualifying volume, but one has to consider what constitutes a "hard" set or a valid set. *Monthly Applications in Strength Sports (MASS)* newsletter research review authors Eric Helms, Mike Zourdos, and Greg Nuckols have discussed (Zourdos 2018) that "hard" could mean a rating of perceived exertion (RPE) of at least six to seven, or three to four reps in reserve (RIR). This means that if you are prescribed to perform a set of eight reps, you could have done 11 or 12 reps if you took it to your limit, but you did eight. This would be considered at the lower end of a hard set. As a guideline or rule of thumb, a hard set would consist of an RIR of zero to four for a given rep count. Later, we will discuss RPE and RIR in greater detail.

Many authors have recently proposed that volume is the primary driver of hypertrophy. This may be true, but context is critical in stating and understanding this statement. Volume is perhaps the key variable (as we must do enough work), but it has little relevance without qualifying it with regard to intensity and effort. Otherwise, the highest volume endurance activities would be the best way to get bigger muscles, and we know that this is not the case.

Before simply adding more work in terms of sets on a given day for a client, you must first consider the following:

- Is the training effective and is the client utilizing sound exercise technique?
- Is the client focused and striving to lift more weight or to do more reps on a regular basis?
- Is the client consistent with training?

Once a client has effective and technically sound exercise form performed with appropriate intensity on a regular basis, then volume may be added. Doing more work can't replace effectiveness, quality of effort, or regularity. Adding training hours does not always equate to more results. The client has to do a sufficient volume of work, not as much as she or he can possibly cram in. If and when training time is added, it should be done very progressively over time.

Now that we have a working concept of why volume is important for hypertrophy, let's take a look at how the practitioner would apply it to hypertrophy programming.

How Much Weekly Volume?

A set volume research meta-analysis by Schoenfeld, Ogborn, and Krieger (2017) has suggested a guideline for number of weekly sets to be 10 to 20+ hard sets per muscle group or movement pattern for hypertrophy, and this appears to be a good rule of thumb. The ballpark number of 10 sets is consistent with what we have experienced as a decent dosage.

The weekly set work set volume is what appears to matter most. What we mean by this is that spreading the training volume across multiple sessions appears to be superior to trying to do it all in one day. As mentioned in our discussion about frequency, several studies have shown superior lean body-mass gains when spreading it out across the week, because intensity and quality will be sacrificed trying to do it all in one session.

Another win for full-body training for the average person!

How Many Sets Per Exercise?

How many sets should you perform per exercise? Again, this depends on the rep range and the training time available. In practice, we typically utilize between one to five sets of an exercise, such as in the following few examples for hypertrophy purposes. These are the same guidelines used in our programming for fat-loss clients because what builds muscle is also what keeps muscle.

1 to 2 sets, 15 reps
3 to 4 sets, 8 reps
3 sets, 12 reps
4 to 5 sets, 4 reps

How Many Reps for Hypertrophy?

There has been a lot of research confirming that low reps (Schoenfeld et al. 2014, 2015) are optimal for strength development. Strength (in terms of 1 Rep Max) has been shown best built in the 1 to 5 rep range with appropriate intensities. This is very clearly the case and will be discussed further in the next chapter. The traditional hypertrophy range is typically prescribed to be 6 to 15 (or up to 20) reps. So, we have the following:

- *Rep range for strength*: 1 to 5 reps
- *Rep range for hypertrophy*: 6 to 20 reps

These can also be correlated to times since reps performed are just a measure of the total time under tension; time under tension is one of the factors that determines the training stimulus. Eight reps performed in 20 seconds is an entirely different training stimulus than 8 reps in 40 seconds. So rather than just selecting a rep range, determine your desired training effect and select a repetition bracket to suit your goals. The following are some generalities:

- *1 to 20 seconds*: Strength development (typically 1 to 5 reps)
- *20 to 40 seconds*: Strength/hypertrophy (typically 5 to 8 reps)
- *40 to 70 seconds*: Hypertrophy development (8 to 15 reps)
- *70 to 120 seconds*: Muscular endurance/stability/metabolic training (15 reps and above).

Research over the past several years has shown that there is not a specific hypertrophy range, so to speak, meaning that if you branch outside the above numbers, you can still get comparable hypertrophy. Dr. Schoenfeld's research (Schoenfeld et al. 2015) has shown that several different rep ranges (and intensities) can lead to similar levels of muscle hypertrophy. Lower reps (5 sec and less) of an adequate number of sets, and higher rep sets than the typical hypertrophy ranges taken to failure (provided the load intensity is not too low) can lead to similar levels of hypertrophy. However, it takes quite a lot of sets to accomplish this with low reps (thus a lot of training time) and conversely, it is physically and mentally fatiguing to take super high rep sets to failure on a regular basis. The traditional hypertrophy rep range may not be the be-all and end-all, but it is a very time-efficient way to get a lot of quality work done with appreciable loads. It ends up being a very practical method for doing hypertrophy work because it is a convenient way to accumulate training volume without taking too long (recall that time is always a limiting factor), creating excessive fatigue, and excessive mental taxation. So even though it is not a hard-and-fast rule, the hypertrophy rep range remains a useful guideline when programming in the real world.

If the goal is only hypertrophy, would staying in the hypertrophy rep range be the best choice in regard to rep selection (which affects load by default)? Actually no; once you advance, you experience the best gains when using a mixture of both higher and lower reps. Basically, the lower reps allow heavier weights to be used, so you are stronger when you return to your original "hypertrophy" rep bracket. If you go higher, you experience a longer time under tension and therefore have more endurance when you return to the original rep bracket. The underlying message is obvious, variety alone can accelerate your progress, and regardless of your goal, the main premise is that it is not merely which rep brackets to use, but also how long to stay within each rep bracket. You will see this in practice with the daily undulating periodization concept in the advanced programming phase.

How Much Load?

Load, often used interchangeably with intensity, is typically understood to be the weight being used. When we say, "How much load?" You usually know what we are talking about. The term *intensity* is often misperceived. Much like any discussion about volume, the first question that needs to be asked when discussing intensity should be: "What do you mean by intensity?"

Intensity of Load

Intensity of load is expressed as a percentage of one repetition maximum, meaning the most weight a person could lift for one repetition of a particular movement (1RM). This is the traditional exercise physiology definition used in studies. It can also be used to refer to the weight being utilized, which is why load and intensity are often used interchangeably. The percentage of 1RM corresponds to a maximum number of repetitions associated with it (see table 5.1).

Table 5.1 Relationship Between %1RM and Maximum Number of Repetitions Performed

Percentage of 1RM	Rep max (RM)
100%	1RM
95%	2RM
90%	3RM-4RM
85%	5RM-6RM
80%	6RM-8RM
75%	8RM-10RM
70%	10RM-12RM
65%	12RM-15RM

Intensity of Effort

Intensity of effort means how hard it is *relatively*, or how hard it is relative to the number of reps being performed, expressed as RPE or RIR. Our colleague Joel Sanders from EXOS also refers to intensity of effort as *intensiveness* to distinguish it from intensity.

We have found RPE (or RIR) to be useful to describe and communicate effort level in a particular set, and these terms can also be used to prescribe loads to a degree. The credit for popularizing RPE in resistance training populations goes to renowned powerlifting coach Mike Tuchscherer of Reactive Training Systems. Dr. Mike Zourdos and Dr. Eric Helms have also conducted considerable research into the use of RPE in resistance-trained populations to help to validate its use.

The chart and descriptions from powerlifter Mike Tuchscherer shown in figure 5.1 is a very helpful tool for choosing loads and rating the perceived exertion in a set. In our experience, the loading chart doesn't work as well with beginners and is more suited to those with a bit of training experience. However, the descriptions of RPE and RIR work pretty well with almost anyone.

Confusion often arises when we use the descriptors of *heavy* and *hard*, as well. It's helpful to think of intensity of load as being a measure of how heavy something is and intensity of effort to be a descriptor of how hard a set of reps feels. Heavy and hard are not interchangeable and should be differentiated when communicating about intensity.

Either of these terms can be applied to hypertrophy training but in our programming we tend to focus on the intensity of effort in regard to the number of reps performed. For hypertrophy training in particular, the reps will dictate the weight in most instances (speed and power work would be a notable exception of course). If we want you to perform six reps we expect you to choose a weight that will be appropriately challenging for six reps. Remember the guideline regarding "hard" sets. Similarly, if we assign a rep bracket of 20 reps, we still expect you to choose a challenging load. A lot of beginners go wrong here by following the typical light weight and high rep nonsense and use five-pound dumbbells for sets of 15 when they are capable of using 30-pound dumbbells for a challenging set of 15. The load selected for the sets of 15 is lighter relative to the load selected for the sets of 6, but this doesn't mean the set of 15 is easy. In most instances, you should not be able to perform many more reps at your given weight.

The most important training principle (regardless of goal) is employing progressive overload. If you do not apply an overload to your body, there is no reason for your

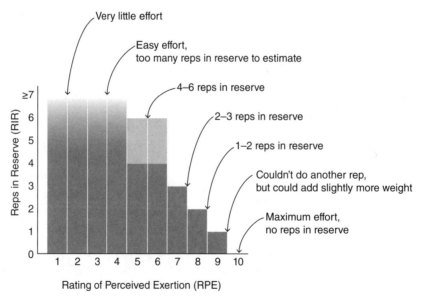

Figure 5.1   Rating of Perceived Exertion (RPE) Chart

Adapted from M.C. Zourdos, A. Klemp, C. Dolan, et al., "Novel Resistance Training-Specific Rating of Perceived Exertion Scale Measuring Repetitions in Reserve," *Journal of Strength Condition and Research* 30, no. 1 (2016): 267-275.

body to make any adaptations. Bottom line, regardless of rep bracket, choose a challenging or appropriate load.

Muscle Building Programming

We will once again give you two phases of a beginner to intermediate program and then provide two phases of a more advanced program. The programs that follow focus on the use of multijoint compound exercises that utilize the most muscle mass. This gives us a lot of bang for our training buck in terms of efficiently building muscle. We always need to remember that approximately 70 percent of our muscle mass is in our back and legs so it is important to train movements that exploit this if we are trying to get bigger. Many of the chosen exercises also allow us to use substantial loads so that we place a good amount of mechanical tension on the muscles involved to create a strong growth adaptation.

In terms of our how we have periodized our rep programming, we have selected a linear periodization scheme for the beginner to intermediate phases and a daily undulating rep scheme for the advanced phases. Linear periodization tends to work well for beginner trainees because they don't need a lot of repetition variability right away, and it also makes load selection less challenging for the coach. We also start with higher reps in the first phase to build potential connective tissue strength and provide what periodization expert Tudor Bompa might call "anatomical adaptation." We accumulate a lot of rep volume in phase 1 which serves as a foundation for phase 2.

For more advanced trainees we move to an undulating rep programming scheme. Advanced trainees need more variability than novices, but that doesn't necessarily mean massive exercise variation. We believe that the body accommodates to the number of reps the fastest, so this is the primary variable we manipulate to provide a different stressor as our training age advances. Since advanced trainees have more training experience and skill in performing exercises (less technical breakdown than beginners), the coach has data that can be used to select loads for the rep targets that are prescribed.

As in the previous chapter, let's explain the actual programming for hypertrophy.

Beginner to Intermediate Program

As in chapter 4, this program is designed to be used by those clients that scored below 15 on our training age rubric that we discussed in chapter 2. Again, it will still work for those who scored over 15, so it wouldn't be wrong to start here with anyone who has the primary goal of hypertrophy. In our experience (and this applies to all programs in this book), an advanced program won't work for a beginner, but a beginner's program will still work, to a degree, for someone who is advanced. Always be sure that selected exercises are a fit for the person in front of you, and refer to the tools in chapter 3 to make necessary adjustments.

The client will alternate between session A and session B on each training day, performing session A six times and session B six times in each phase. Phases 1 and 2 are each designed to be done for four to six weeks, depending on how frequently the client trains each week. This also provides some flexibility. If the client trains with a frequency of three times per week, which we would suggest as being optimal (see table 5.2), phases 1 and 2 will be completed in four weeks. If the client trains two times per week (see table 5.3), each phase will be completed in six weeks. After completing all of the A and B sessions for phase 1, the client moves on to phase 2. See tables 5.4 through 5.7 for the example beginner to intermediate muscle-building program (the tempo key is on page 29).

Table 5.2   Beginner to Intermediate Phase 1 and 2 Sample Weekly Schedule: Three Sessions per Week

	Mon	Tues	Wed	Thurs	Fri	Sat	Sun
Week 1	Session A		Session B		Session A		
Week 2	Session B		Session A		Session B		
Week 3	Session A		Session B		Session A		
Week 4	Session B		Session A		Session B		

Table 5.3   Beginner to Intermediate Phase 1 and 2 Sample Weekly Schedule: Two Sessions per Week

	Mon	Tues	Wed	Thurs	Fri	Sat	Sun
Week 1	Session A			Session B			
Week 2	Session A			Session B			
Week 3	Session A			Session B			
Week 4	Session A			Session B			
Week 5	Session A			Session B			
Week 6	Session A			Session B			

Table 5.4   Beginner to Intermediate Muscle-Building Program: Phase 1, Day A

Core training			SETS	REPS	TEMPO	REST
	1a.	Front plank	1-2	1	30-45 sec	N/A
	1b.	Cable tall-kneeling antirotation press	1-2	10 each side	1-3-1	60 sec
Resistance training			SETS	REPS	TEMPO	REST
	2a.	Goblet squat	2-3	12-15	—	60 sec
	2b.	Dumbbell three-point neutral-grip row	2-3	12-15 each side	Mod	60 sec
	3a.	One-dumbbell staggered-stance Romanian deadlift	2-3	12 each side	—	60 sec
	3b.	Push-up	2-3	12	Mod	60 sec

Table 5.5   Beginner to Intermediate Muscle-Building Program: Phase 1, Day B

Core training			SETS	REPS	TEMPO	REST
	1a.	Sandbag full dead bug with alternating leg reach	1-2	5 each side	FE	N/A
	1b.	Side plank from knees	1-2	4-6 each side	5 sec	60 sec
Resistance training			SETS	REPS	TEMPO	REST
	2a.	Dumbbell Romanian deadlift	2-3	12-15	Mod	60 sec
	2b.	Kettlebell half-kneeling single-arm overhead press	2-3	12-15 each side	Mod	60 sec
	3a.	Goblet split squat	2-3	12 each side	—	60 sec
	3b.	Kneeling neutral-grip pulldown	2-3	12-15	Mod	60 sec

Table 5.6 Beginner to Intermediate Muscle-Building Program: Phase 2, Day A

Core training			SETS	REPS	TEMPO	REST
	1a.	Suspension trainer front plank	1-2	1	30-45 sec	N/A
	1b.	Cable bar half-kneeling chop	1-2	8 each side	Slow	60 sec
Resistance training			SETS	REPS	TEMPO	REST
	2.	Front squat	2-3	8	—	2 min+
	3a.	Cable seated neutral-grip row	2-3	8-10	Mod	60 sec
	3b.	One-dumbbell block single-leg deadlift	2-3	10 each	—	60 sec
	4a.	Dumbbell neutral-grip bench press	2-3	8-10	Mod	60 sec
	4b.	Rope split-stance neutral-grip face pull with external rotation	2	10-12	Mod	60 sec

Table 5.7 Beginner to Intermediate Muscle-Building Program: Phase 2, Day B

Core training			SETS	REPS	TEMPO	REST
	1a.	Sandbag full dead bug with alternating arm and leg reach	1-2	5 each side	FE	0 sec
	1b.	Side plank	1-2	4-6 each side	5 sec	60 sec
Resistance training			SETS	REPS	TEMPO	REST
	2.	High hex bar deadlift	2-3	8	—	2 min +
	3a.	Suspension trainer inverted neutral-grip row	2-3	8-10	Mod	60 sec
	3b.	Goblet rear-foot-elevated split squat	2-3	10 each side	—	60 sec
	4a.	Two-dumbbell overhead press	2-3	8-10	Mod	60 sec
	4b.	Swiss ball supine hip extension leg curl	2	8-10	Slow	60 sec

Advanced Program

This program is designed to be used by clients with a primary goal of hypertrophy who scored 15 points or above on our training age rubric discussed in chapter 2. It should not be used by clients who scored less than 15 points.

The client will alternate between session A and session B on each training day. Take note of the repetition changes on each of the training days. The client will perform session A six times and session B six times in each phase. Phases 1 and 2 are each designed to be done for four to six weeks, depending on how frequently the client trains each week. This also provides some flexibility. If the client trains with a frequency of three times per week (see table 5.8), phases 1 and 2 will each be completed in four weeks, and if training two times per week (see table 5.9), it will take six weeks to complete each phase. See tables 5.10 through 5.13 for the sample advanced muscle-building program.

Table 5.8 Advanced Phase 1 and 2 Sample Weekly Schedule: Three Sessions per Week

	Mon	Tues	Wed	Thurs	Fri	Sat	Sun
Week 1	Session A (10 reps)		Session B (5 reps)		Session A (15 reps)		
Week 2	Session B (10 reps)		Session A (5 reps)		Session B (15 reps)		
Week 3	Session A (10 reps)		Session B (5 reps)		Session A (15 reps)		
Week 4	Session B (10 reps)		Session A (5 reps)		Session B (15 reps)		

Table 5.9 Advanced Phase 1 and 2 Sample Weekly Schedule: Two Sessions per Week

	Mon	Tues	Wed	Thurs	Fri	Sat	Sun
Week 1	Session A (10 reps)			Session B (5 reps)			
Week 2	Session A (15 reps)			Session B (10 reps)			
Week 3	Session A (5 reps)			Session B (15 reps)			
Week 4	Session A (10 reps)			Session B (5 reps)			
Week 5	Session A (15 reps)			Session B (10 reps)			
Week 6	Session A (5 reps)			Session B (15 reps)			

Table 5.10 Advanced Muscle-Building Program: Phase 1, Day A

Core training			SETS	REPS	TEMPO	REST
	1.	Suspension trainer kneeling fallout	2-3	6-8	Slow	60 sec
Combination or power development			SETS	REPS	TEMPO	REST
	2.	Box jump	3-4	4	X	30 sec
Resistance training			SETS	REPS	TEMPO	REST
	3a.	Back squat				
		Sessions 1 & 4	2-3	10	—	60 sec
		Sessions 2 & 5	2	15	—	60 sec
		Sessions 3 & 6	4	5	—	90 sec
	3b.	Chin-up				
		Sessions 1 & 4	2-3	10	Mod	60 sec
		Sessions 2 & 5	2	15	—	60 sec
		Sessions 3 & 6	4	5	Mod	90 sec

		SETS	REPS	TEMPO	REST
4a.	One-dumbbell single-leg Romanian deadlift				
	Sessions 1 & 4	2-3	10 each side	—	60 sec
	Sessions 2 & 5	2	15 each side	—	60 sec
	Sessions 3 & 6	4	5 each side	—	90 sec
4b.	Dumbbell low-incline bench press				
	Sessions 1 & 4	2-3	10	—	60 sec
	Sessions 2 & 5	2	15	—	60 sec
	Sessions 3 & 6	4	5	—	90 sec

Table 5.11   Advanced Muscle-Building Program: Phase 1, Day B

Core training		SETS	REPS	TEMPO	REST
	1. Suspension trainer side plank	2-3	1 each side	20-30 sec	60 sec
Combination or power development		SETS	REPS	TEMPO	REST
	2. Cable rotational low-to-high lift	2	8 each side	—	60 sec
Resistance training		SETS	REPS	TEMPO	REST
	3a. Deadlift				
	Sessions 1 & 4	3-4	5	—	90 sec
	Sessions 2 & 5	3	10	—	60 sec
	Sessions 3 & 6	2	15	—	60 sec
	3b. Barbell overhead press				
	Sessions 1 & 4	3-4	5	Mod	90 sec
	Sessions 2 & 5	3	10	Mod	60 sec
	Sessions 3 & 6	2	15	Mod	60 sec
	4a. Two-dumbbell reverse lunge				
	Sessions 1 & 4	3-4	5 each side	—	90 sec
	Sessions 2 & 5	3	10 each side	—	60 sec
	Sessions 3 & 6	2	15 each side	—	60 sec
	4b. Cable seated neutral-grip row				
	Sessions 1 & 4	3-4	5	Mod	90 sec
	Sessions 2 & 5	3	10	Mod	60 sec
	Sessions 3 & 6	2	15	Mod	60 sec

Table 5.12   Advanced Muscle-Building Program: Phase 2, Day A

Core training			SETS	REPS	TEMPO	REST
	1.	Ab wheel roll-out	2-3	5-7	Slow	60 sec
Combination or power development			SETS	REPS	TEMPO	REST
	2.	Kettlebell swing	3-4	10	X	45 sec
Resistance training			SETS	REPS	TEMPO	REST
	3a.	Back squat with pause				
		Sessions 1 & 4	2-3	12	—	60 sec
		Sessions 2 & 5	4	4	Mod	90 sec
		Sessions 3 & 6	3	8	Mod	60 sec
	3b.	Dumbbell bench row				
		Sessions 1 & 4	2-3	12	Mod	60 sec
		Sessions 2 & 5	4	4	Mod	90 sec
		Sessions 3 & 6	3	8	Mod	60 sec
	4a.	Two-dumbbell single-leg Romanian deadlift				
		Sessions 1 & 4	2-3	12 each side	—	60 sec
		Sessions 2 & 5	4	4 each side	—	90 sec
		Sessions 3 & 6	3	8 each side	—	60 sec
	4b.	Barbell bench press				
		Sessions 1 & 4	2-3	12	—	60 sec
		Sessions 2 & 5	4	4	Mod	90 sec
		Sessions 3 & 6	3	8	Mod	60 sec

Table 5.13   Advanced Muscle-Building Program: Phase 2, Day B

Core training			SETS	REPS	TEMPO	REST
	1.	Side plank + cable single-arm row	2-3	8 each side	Slow	60 sec
Combination or power development			SETS	REPS	TEMPO	REST
	2.	Turkish get-up	2	1 each side	—	60 sec
Resistance training			SETS	REPS	TEMPO	REST
	3a.	Snatch-grip deadlift				
		Sessions 1 & 4	3-4	4	—	90 sec
		Sessions 2 & 5	3	8	—	60 sec
		Sessions 3 & 6	3	12	—	60 sec
	3b.	Barbell push press				
		Sessions 1 & 4	3-4	4	—	90 sec
		Sessions 2 & 5	3	8	—	60 sec
		Sessions 3 & 6	3	12	—	60 sec
	4a.	Two-dumbbell front-foot-elevated reverse lunge				
		Sessions 1 & 4	3-4	4 each side	—	90 sec
		Sessions 2 & 5	3	8 each side	—	60 sec
		Sessions 3 & 6	3	12 each side	—	60 sec
	4b.	Pull-up				
		Sessions 1 & 4	3-4	4	—	90 sec
		Sessions 2 & 5	3	8	—	60 sec
		Sessions 3 & 6	3	12	—	60 sec

CABLE TALL-KNEELING ANTIROTATION PRESS

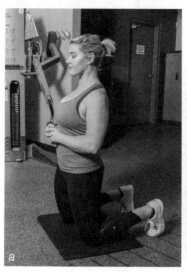 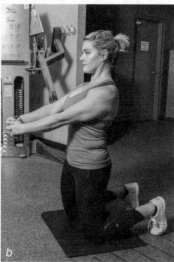

Setup and Performance

- Set the pulley to about midchest when in a tall-kneeling (both knees down) position.
- In the tall-kneeling position, turn perpendicular to the pulley holding the handle with the outside hand. The inside hand will overlap it.
- The handle is positioned just below the sternum touching the body.
- Press the handle straight out from the body, pause, and then return the handle back to the starting point just below the sternum. Repeat.

Key Performance Points

- Be sure to keep the torso stacked through the whole movement. Keep the rib cage stacked over the hips. Think of this as a half-kneeling plank.
- Fully extend the elbows when pressing out and keep the handle directly in line with the middle of body. Imagine you are cutting the body into an equal left and right half with the handle.
- Drive through the ground with the toes so it helps to stabilize the middle as well as engage the glutes.
- Make sure you fully extend the arms when pressing out.

DUMBBELL THREE-POINT NEUTRAL-GRIP ROW

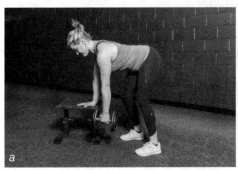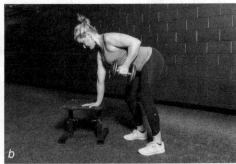

Setup and Performance

- Stand in front of an 18-inch-high (46 cm) bench or box. Hinge over at the hip and place a hand on the bench as a point of support.
- The feet are placed about shoulder-width apart and away from the bench.
- Pick up a dumbbell in one hand. The back will be relatively flat like a tabletop.
- Pull the dumbbell back toward the side and bottom of the rib cage.
- Pause, return to the extended arm position, and repeat.

Key Performance Points

- When rowing ensure that the shoulder blade is moving. A common error is to only bend the elbow without much shoulder blade movement. A good cue for all rowing-type movement is to "spread the logo on the front of your t-shirt."
- The upper arm may go past the torso as long as it doesn't move much past the shoulder blade.
- Bring the dumbbell toward the bottom of the rib cage, not into the armpit. A good position to have at the top of the movement is an "open" elbow angle of about 90 degrees.
- Keep the spine relatively straight and stable.

KETTLEBELL HALF-KNEELING
SINGLE-ARM OVERHEAD PRESS

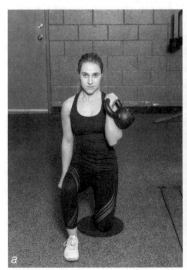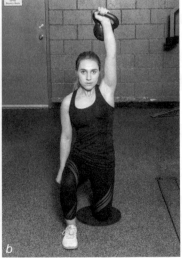

Setup and Performance

- Begin in a half-kneeling position with one kettlebell in the front rack position.
- The kettlebell will be held on the "rear leg" side.
- Press the kettlebell up to the top position with the palm facing out.
- Pull the bell back down into the rack position and repeat.

Key Performance Points

- Keep the wrist neutral and flat.
- Make sure that the pressing arm is straight at the top and vertical from all angles.
- Ensure that the back knee, hip, and shoulder are relatively stacked, or lined up, when viewed from the side.

ONE-DUMBBELL BLOCK SINGLE-LEG DEADLIFT

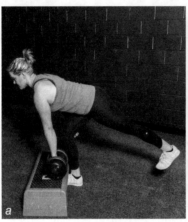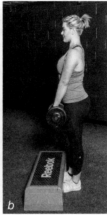

Setup and Performance

- Set up a block or sturdy step that allows the feet to be slightly underneath it and place a dumbbell on the block.
- Stand on one leg facing the step with the foot under the step.
- Hip-hinge on one leg pushing the hip back and bending forward.
- Reach down to grip the dumbbell with the opposite hand (if you are standing on the right foot, you will hold the dumbbell with the left hand). This is a contra-loaded position because it is held in the hand that is opposite the working leg.
- Keep the shoulders square at the bottom, create tension and "push" the slack out of the dumbbell BEFORE attempting to lift it.
- Push the floor away and stand upright pulling up the dumbbell in a straight line.
- Reverse the motion, and reset on the block.

Key Performance Points

- We recommend that you use a sturdy step for this exercise.
- This version provides a second point of contact to stabilize at the bottom of the movement.
- Be sure to keep the stance or working leg bent at the bottom of the movement. This is critical as it allows the hips to move back properly; if the hips don't move back they will spin open and balance will be compromised.
- Keep the spine stable and in a relatively straight line during the movement.

ROPE SPLIT-STANCE NEUTRAL-GRIP FACE PULL WITH EXTERNAL ROTATION

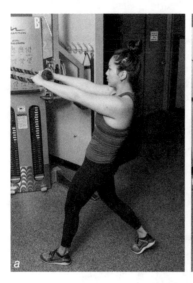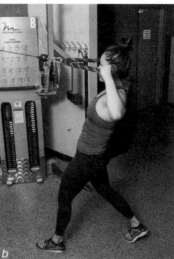

Setup and Performance

- Set up a pulley to a bit higher than head height with a long "triceps" rope handle attached to it.
- Grab toward the end of the rope with the thumbs turned back toward the body and get into a long split stance with the arms straight.
- Initiate the movement with the shoulder blades and pull the rope back in the direction of the eyes.
- With the hands above the elbows in the finish position, pause for a count, and spread the rope slightly.
- Return to the starting position and repeat.

Key Performance Points

- Hold up the upper arms so that they form about 90-degree angles at the finish position.
- When viewed from the side, the hands and elbows should be relatively even with each other at the finish position.

SANDBAG FULL DEAD BUG
WITH ALTERNATING ARM AND LEG REACH

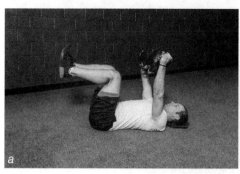 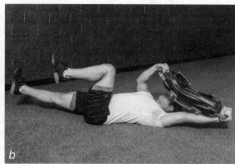

Setup and Performance

- Lie on the back and bring the legs up into a 90-degree flexed position.
- Hold the sandbag by the outside handles over the chest with the wrists straight and arms fully extended.
- Pull the handles of the bag apart and bring the ribs down to slightly press the low back into the floor.
- Maintaining pelvic position, extend one leg so that it hovers slightly off the ground.
- Simultaneously, as the leg extends, reach back toward the ground with the opposing arm.
- Fully exhale at this position. Simultaneously bring the arms and legs back to the starting position and repeat on the other side.

Key Performance Points

- Be sure to pull the handles of the sandbag apart while extending the leg. This will help to create and maintain top-down body tension and pelvic stability. Prevent the bag from sagging.
- Reset the tension between each rep.

SWISS BALL SUPINE HIP EXTENSION LEG CURL

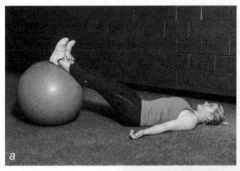 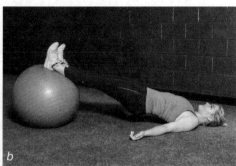

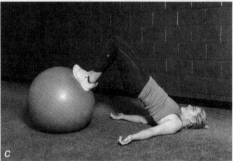

Setup and Performance

- Lie on the floor facing up with the legs straight and the heels placed together on top of a Swiss ball. The arms are at the sides with the palms up.
- Set the core and lift the hips up so that the body forms a straight line from the shoulder, hips, knees, and ankles.
- While keeping the hip extended, flex the knee joint pulling the ball in toward the butt.
- Slowly return to the starting position and repeat.

Key Performance Point

- The hips should rise while the knee joint flexes. For every inch (3 cm) the shoes come back, the belt line raises an inch so that the hips stay extended. We want the hip extended while the knees flex.

ADVANCED MUSCLE-BUILDING PROGRAM EXERCISES

SUSPENSION TRAINER KNEELING FALLOUT

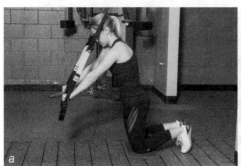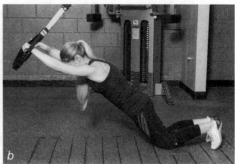

Setup and Performance

- Set the suspension trainer to the fully lengthened position.
- Kneel down on both knees with the knees about hip-width apart facing away from the anchor point with the hips extended holding onto the handles with the straight arms. The knees, hips, and shoulder are in a straight line with the arms out in front of you.
- While keeping the kneeling plank position of the torso, move the torso and hips toward the ground while raising the arms up to a position where the arms are almost in line with the head.
- Maintaining the solid plank position, push back into the tall-kneeling setup.

Key Performance Points

- Start with a conservative body angle. The further behind the anchor point you move the knees, the more challenging the fallout becomes.
- Keep the shoulders "sucked" into the sockets to maintain tension.
- Keep the ribs and hips together as you move the arm forward. This is an exercise that should *not* be felt in the lumbar spine.

ONE-DUMBBELL SINGLE-LEG ROMANIAN DEADLIFT

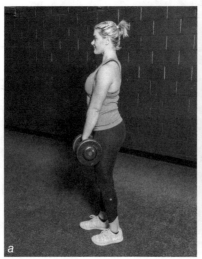 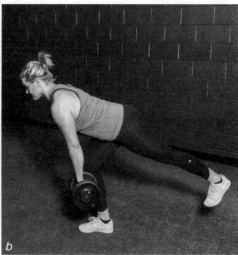

Setup and Performance

- Stand upright and pick up one foot. The dumbbell will be held on the same side as the leg that is going back.
- Hip-hinge on the working leg while the rear leg moves back. A straight line should be formed from the rear leg to the head.
- The dumbbell lowers in a straight line to a position that is somewhere between the level of the bottom of the knee and midshin.
- Push the floor away and hip-hinge to return to the starting position while pulling the dumbbell up in a straight line. Repeat.

Key Performance Points

- This is an RDL, meaning you start at the top of the lift and push the hips backward. The front shin angle will be relatively vertical.
- Keep the spine stable, and move through the hips. Be sure to establish this position at the beginning, before the lift begins.
- Be sure to keep the working leg bent at the bottom of the movement. This is critical because it allows the hips to move back properly; if the hips don't move back, they will spin open and balance will be compromised.
- Keep the shoulders square at the bottom.

CABLE ROTATIONAL LOW-TO-HIGH LIFT

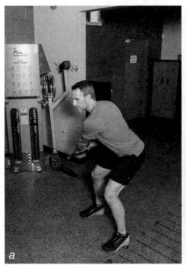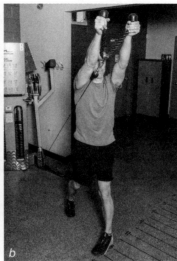

Setup and Performance

- Attach a "triceps" rope to the low pulley of the machine.
- Stand sideways to the pulley with the feet a bit wider than shoulder-width apart and the hips pushed back holding the rope toward the ends with the thumbs up.
- Sit back and slightly down while turning the shoulders perpendicular to the hips. The cable will be across the body.
- Strongly drive the floor away while rotating, and pull the rope to the body and then press the rope up in a diagonal motion.
- Reverse the motion and return to the starting position, reset, and repeat.

Key Performance Points

- The rotation occurs in the upper back and the hips, not the lumbar spine.
- Be sure to turn the shoulders perpendicular to the hips in the starting position.
- Don't try to hold a long static pause in the finish position.

TWO-DUMBBELL FRONT-FOOT-ELEVATED REVERSE LUNGE

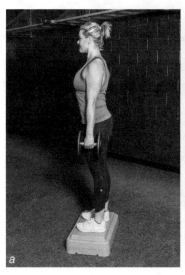 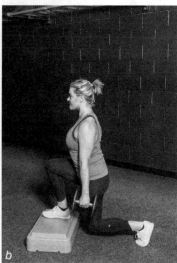

Setup and Performance

- Stand on a solid elevated surface (stacked mats or a sturdy step) that is about four to six inches (10-15 cm) high with the feet about hip-width apart with a dumbbell in each hand.
- Step back off the surface with one foot into a lunge with the back knee almost touching the floor, and then push through the front foot and return to the starting position.
- Repeat for the designated number of reps on each leg.

Key Performance Points

- Having the front foot elevated allows for a greater range of motion and a deep lunge position.
- Ensure that the back knee, hip, and shoulder are relatively stacked at the bottom position of each lunge. A slight forward lean is fine as long as one stays stacked as described.
- The trailing leg's knee should not bang on the floor, it should almost touch the floor.
- Brace the abs to keep the pelvis stable during the lunge.

CHAPTER 6

Strength-Building Programs

Strength comes in many forms; therefore, we need a working definition of *strength*. We can, once again, ask the clarifying question: "What do you mean by strong?" One of the best definitions of strength comes from StrongFirst founder Pavel Tsatsouline. In his book *The Naked Warrior* (2003), Pavel defines strength as the ability to generate force under given conditions—a simple and concise definition with a broad application. The qualifier of "given conditions" is key here. When most people refer to strength, they are referring to maximal strength, which is typically measured by the most weight you can lift for one repetition in a given movement. Keep in mind that strength doesn't mean 1RM maximum only. Getting stronger in any rep range is still getting stronger.

At our gym, we often use the "rope ladder analogy"[1] to illustrate why strength is so important (see figure 6.1). Imagine if we place the quality of maximal strength on the top rung of a hypothetical rope ladder. We can now place all other physical qualities and attributes, such as power, speed, agility, and endurance, on each of the subsequent lower rungs. Endurance would go on the very bottom rung.

Now, if we leave maximal strength on the top rung of the ladder and try to push up directly on any of the lower rungs, we quickly find that we have a limited amount of space available before we run into the rung above it. At some point, we can no longer push that one rung any higher. The ladder simply won't go any higher. If we only push on the bottom rung (endurance), we very quickly run into the rung above it without causing any movement at all in any of the other rungs above it. However, if we push up on our top rung, all the other rungs follow and every rung on the ladder is raised higher. This is how maximal strength affects all of the other physical preparation qualities, and it is the reason why this top rung of strength is so foundational.

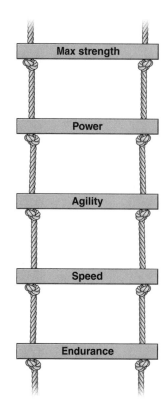

Figure 6.1 Rope ladder analogy to illustrate the importance of strength.

---

[1] Credit for this analogy goes to Charles Staley, who wrote about it in an article on *T-Nation.com*.

Improving Strength = Improving Force Production

Getting stronger is about improving force production. Briefly, here are two of the primary ways that muscles produce force.

- *Neuromuscular efficiency*: The coordinated actions of all the muscle groups in a particular movement through intramuscular coordination (i.e., motor unit recruitment, rate coding, or motor unit firing rate) and intermuscular coordination.
- *Muscular cross-sectional area*: The increased size of the contractile tissues (hypertrophy).

Strength is typically qualified in two primary ways: *absolute strength* and *relative strength*. Both are important in life and in athletics, and can be measured by simply tracking training loads. Absolute strength is a measure of overall strength, or force exerted, regardless of bodyweight. For example, a person that squats one rep of 500 pounds (227 kg) is stronger than a person who squats one rep of 400 pounds (181 kg) in terms of absolute weight lifted. Relative strength is a measure of overall strength, or force exerted, relative to the individual's bodyweight. Using the previous example, let's say the person who squats 500 pounds weighs 300 pounds (136 kg), and the person who squats 400 pounds weighs 200 pounds (91 kg). The 500-pound squatter performs a 1.67-times-bodyweight squat, and the 400-pound squatter performs a 2-times-bodyweight squat. Therefore, relative to their bodyweight, the 400-pound squatter is stronger.

Let's look at another interesting example using the same two people. Let's say our 300-pound (136 kg) person can perform three bodyweight pull-ups, and our 200-pound (91 kg) person can perform the same three bodyweight pull-ups with an additional 50 pounds (23 kg). Who is stronger in an absolute sense? At first glance one might think the person using the additional 50 pounds is stronger because they are using additional load, but if we look closer, our 300-pound person is actually stronger in this exercise *absolutely* because this person is using more total weight (300 lb vs. 250 lb [113 kg]).

That said, we are not saying strength alone is the be-all and end-all of a complete training program, but if we prioritize, strength is the most important limiting factor if we determine it to be lacking. If all other things are equal, being strong raises the whole ladder higher giving a bigger bang for the training buck.

Key Variables in Strength Programming

Next, we discuss the key variables involved in getting stronger and how they apply to the development of strength as a primary goal. We also show how to measure strength against various standards to determine general standings.

Sets, Reps, and Intensity

Some of the research meta-analyses (Ralston et al. 2017) have shown that for strength, between 5 to 12 sets of an exercise per week will lead to strength development. It must be reiterated that this is a guideline and not a rule, but it provides rough numbers to use, and one should be aware of extremes that widely vary from this range.

As mentioned briefly in chapter 4, there has been a considerable amount of research showing that low reps are clearly optimal for maximal strength development. Strength (in terms of 1RM) is best gained in the 1 to 5 rep range with appropriate intensities. This intensity is typically around 80 percent of 1RM and higher. Once again, these are guidelines and not hard cut-off points. You can obviously still gain strength (in terms of 1RM) with reps that are a bit higher and intensity that is slightly lower. Completely untrained lifters can get strong with loads that are even quite a bit lower. Generally, the more advanced is the athlete, the higher the intensities that must be used. Practicing the skill of lifting heavy weights is one of the best ways to improve neuromuscular efficiency.

Progressive Overload

Progressive overload applies to both strength and hypertrophy (see chapter 5), and all training, for that matter. To encourage the body to change, new demands or stresses need to be placed upon it. Progressive overload is not a new concept. Many of you have heard the story of Milo of Croton, the Greek wrestler who picked up a baby calf every morning, put it on his shoulders, and carried it. Over the years the calf became a fully-grown bull. Those small increases in the bull's body weight over time allowed Milo to grow bigger and stronger as well, so at the end of his "training," he was able to carry a fully-grown bull. It is not important whether this story is 100 percent true or not (we know strength gain is not linear; otherwise we would all be squatting thousands of pounds by now). What is important is that it illustrates the concept of how progressive overload works.

The human body is essentially resistant to change, or what scientists call homeostasis. Homeostasis is defined scientifically as "the property of a system that regulates its internal environment and tends to maintain a stable, constant condition." (What Is Homeostasis? - Definition & Examples, 2015). This means that the body wants to stay the same: the same temperature, the same weight, the same strength. The body does not want to change. To force a change, we need to apply a new demand or stimulus to overload the body and create a stress that the body is not accustomed to. Hans Selye (1956) used a similar model in what he termed the GAS model, or General Adaptation to Stress. Essentially, after being exposed to stress (the alarm phase) our bodies will upregulate to handle the stressor (the resistance phase), which is really what we are exploiting here. The third phase of Selye's model is exhaustion, which is the reason for periodization and the recovery and regeneration principle. Once the body has adapted to the demands, it must be overloaded again with stress applied in an increasing amount. So, to become stronger or bigger, the weights used need to be increased over time.

The body is smart and constantly adapting; whenever we apply a stimulus, the body adapts. However, if we don't change that stimulus often enough the body becomes stale, gets used to the demands, and stops adapting, leading to no progress. Therefore, the basic premise is to continually increase or change the stress to continue making progress. However, most coaches and trainers tend to only define stress as the "load on the bar." This is short sighted. It may happen because the word *load* is part of the term *progressive overload*, which is a big part, but not all of it. Perhaps we could think of it as progressive stress.

Load is clearly equated with intensity of load (weight being used), and without a doubt, tension overload occurs by increasing the weight used over time, but progressive overload itself can come in various forms. We would be remiss if we did not mention the other ways to provide overload or stress. Not only does the training load need to be progressively increased, but the training stimulus also needs to be periodically varied. This variation also allows us to implement new methods in the program to keep the client's program from becoming stale. We can adjust exercise order, the exercises themselves, sets, reps, rep speed, rest periods, load used, and the implements used (e.g., dumbbells or barbells). It is smart to be aware of and utilize all of the variables when designing programs.

Standards for Strength

In our training age rubric presented in chapter 2 (see question 5 in figure 2.1), we assign some simple numbers to qualify a client's training age on a very rudimentary level. Make no mistake, those earlier numbers given does not necessarily imply strength; the numbers simply help to determine a client's starting point.

We consider the numbers in tables 6.1 and 6.2 to be more representative of solid strength levels for adults (entry-level strength) and athletes (baseline strong). Again, they are not meant to be endpoints (although they can be for certain people) but are provided to give some context. These numbers are compiled from experiences at our gym and from a wide variety of influences including, but not limited to, Pavel and his StrongFirst team, Mike Boyle and his team of coaches, our colleagues Mike Robertson and Eric Cressey, and the author of *Brawn*, Stuart McRobert.

Some of these basic foundational movements are the best way to quantify strength. They aren't fancy or sexy, but they get the job done. There are many more movements to build strength, but they are more difficult to measure and to provide general standards.

Table 6.1   Adult Strength Standards

Movement pattern	Exercise	Females (age: 35-60)	Males (age: 35-60)
Pull	Chin-up	BW, 1 rep	BW, 3-5 reps
	Suspension trainer inverted row	BW with feet elevated 18 in. (46 cm), 1-5 reps	BW with feet elevated 18 in. (46 cm), 5-10 reps
	Dumbbell row	0.25 × BW, 6-8 reps each side	0.4 × BW, 6-8 reps each side
Squat (symmetrical stance)	Back squat	1.0 × BW, 1 rep	1.5 × BW, 1 rep
	Front squat	0.875 × BW, 1 rep	1.125 × BW, 1 rep
Hip hinge	Deadlift	1.125 × BW, 1 rep	1.75 × BW, 1 rep
Push	Push-up	10+ reps	20+ reps
	Bench press	0.6 × BW, 1 rep	1.0 × BW, 1 rep
	Overhead press	0.4 × BW, 1 rep	0.6 × BW, 1 rep
Hip hinge (single-leg)	One-kettlebell or dumbbell single-leg Romanian deadlift	0.4 × BW, 6-8 reps each side	0.5 × BW, 6-8 reps each side
Squat (single-leg)	Single-leg squat from box	BW, 5 reps each side	BW, 5 reps each side
Core	Ab wheel roll-out on knees	BW, 5 reps (full rep is nose near floor)	BW, 5 reps (full rep is nose near floor)

BW = bodyweight

Table 6.2 Athlete Strength Standards

Movement pattern	Exercise	Female	Male
Pull	Chin-up	BW, 5 reps	BW, 10 reps or 0.5 × BW, 1 rep
	Suspension trainer inverted row	BW with feet elevated 18 in. (46 cm), 5-10 reps	BW with feet elevated 18 in. (46 cm), 10-15 reps
	Dumbbell row	0.35 × BW, 6-8 reps each side	0.5 × BW, 6-8 reps each side
Squat (parallel stance)	Back squat	1.5 × BW, 1 rep	2.0 × BW, 1 rep
	Front squat	1.375 × BW, 1 rep	1.625 × BW, 1 rep
Hip hinge (parallel stance)	Deadlift	1.625-2.0 × BW, 1 rep	2.0-2.5 × BW, 1 rep
Push	Bench press	1.0 × BW, 1 rep	1.5 × BW x 1 rep
	Overhead press	0.5-0.6 × BW, 1 rep	0.8-1.0 × BW, 1 rep
	Kettlebell single-arm overhead press	0.33 × BW, 1 rep	0.5 × BW, 1 rep
	Push-up	15+ reps	30 + reps
Hip hinge (single-leg)	One-kettlebell or dumbbell single-leg Romanian deadlift	0.5 × BW, 6-8 reps each side	0.5 × BW, 6-8 reps each side
Squat (single-leg)	Single-leg squat from box	Plus 0.4 × BW, 1 rep each side	Plus 0.5 × BW, 1 rep each side
Squat (split stance)	Barbell reverse lunge or split squat	Plus 0.7 × BW, 5 reps each side	Plus 1.0 × BW, 5 reps each side
	Two-dumbbell rear-foot-elevated split squat	0.4 × BW (each dumbbell), 6 reps each side	0.5 × BW (each dumbbell), 6 reps each side

BW = bodyweight

Strength-Building Programming

We will once again share two phases of a beginner to intermediate program and then provide two phases of a more advanced program. In terms of periodization for the rep programming, again, we selected a linear periodization scheme for the beginner to intermediate phases, and a daily undulating rep scheme for the advanced phases. Linear periodization tends to work well for beginner trainees because they don't need a lot of repetition variability right away, and this also makes load selection less challenging for the coach. In phase 1 of the beginner to intermediate phase we start with 8 rep sets and move to 6 rep sets in phase 2. For more advanced trainees we move to a daily undulating rep programming scheme. Notice that in both phases of our advanced programming, we focus on sets of 3 to 6 reps of the primary exercise on each day to build more maximal strength.

We will use our typical A and B session full-body split for our beginner to intermediate trainees, and a different type of split for our advanced strength phases, which is an A/B/C/D split which hasn't been introduced yet. This advanced strength phase is set up as Hinge/Pull, Squat/Push, Pull/Hinge, and Push/Squat split on each of the respective days. Each day we focus on a primary exercise of either a hinge, squat, pull, or push with a secondary focus that supports the primary one with hypertrophy work. Please refer to tables 10.25 through 10.32 for the details on how this is outlined.

Beginner to Intermediate Program

As in chapter 5, this program is designed to be used by clients who scored below 15 on our training age rubric discussed in chapter 2. It will also work for those who scored over 15 so it wouldn't be wrong to start here with anyone who has the goal of building strength as a primary goal. In either case, be sure that the selected exercises are a fit for the person in front of you, and refer to the tools in chapter 3 to make any adjustments.

The client will alternate between session A and session B on each training day, performing session A six times and session B six times in each phase. Phases 1 and 2 are each designed to be done for four to six weeks, depending on how frequently the client trains each week. This also provides some flexibility. If the client trains with a frequency of three times per week, which we suggest as optimal (see table 6.3), phases 1 and 2 will each be completed in four weeks, and if training two times per week (see table 6.4), it will take six weeks to complete each phase. After completing all of the A and B sessions for phase 1, the client moves on to phase 2. See tables 6.5 through 6.8 for the sample beginner to intermediate strength-building program (the tempo key is on page 29).

Table 6.3 Beginner to Intermediate Phase 1 and 2 Sample Weekly Schedule: Three Sessions per Week

	Mon	Tues	Wed	Thurs	Fri	Sat	Sun
Week 1	Session A		Session B		Session A		
Week 2	Session B		Session A		Session B		
Week 3	Session A		Session B		Session A		
Week 4	Session B		Session A		Session B		

Table 6.4 Beginner to Intermediate Phase 1 and 2 Sample Weekly Schedule: Two Sessions per Week

	Mon	Tues	Wed	Thurs	Fri	Sat	Sun
Week 1	Session A			Session B			
Week 2	Session A			Session B			
Week 3	Session A			Session B			
Week 4	Session A			Session B			
Week 5	Session A			Session B			
Week 6	Session A			Session B			

Table 6.5 Beginner to Intermediate Strength-Building Program: Phase 1, Day A

Core training			SETS	REPS	TEMPO	REST
	1a.	Front plank	1-2	1	30-45 sec	0 sec
	1b.	Cable tall-kneeling antirotation press	1-2	10 each side	1-3-1	60 sec
Resistance training			SETS	REPS	TEMPO	REST
	2a.	Goblet squat with pause	2-3	8	Mod	90 sec
	2b.	Cable kneeling underhand-grip pulldown	2-3	8-10	—	90 sec
	3a.	One-dumbbell staggered-stance Romanian deadlift	2-3	8 each side	—	90 sec
	3b.	Push-up	2-3	8-10	—	90 sec

Table 6.6   Beginner to Intermediate Strength-Building Program: Phase 1, Day B

Core training			SETS	REPS	TEMPO	REST
	1a.	Sandbag dead bug with alternate-leg reach	1-2	5 each side	FE	0 sec
	1b.	Side plank from knees	1-2	4-6 each side	5 sec	60 sec
Resistance training			**SETS**	**REPS**	**TEMPO**	**REST**
	2a.	Barbell Romanian deadlift	2-3	8	—	90 sec
	2b.	Kettlebell single-arm overhead press	2-3	8-10 each side	—	90 sec
	3a.	Goblet split squat	2-3	8 each side	—	90 sec
	3b.	Dumbbell bench neutral-grip row	2-3	8	—	90 sec

Table 6.7   Beginner to Intermediate Strength-Building Program: Phase 2, Day A

Core training			SETS	REPS	TEMPO	REST
	1a.	Suspension trainer front plank	1-2	1	30-45 sec	N/A
	1b.	Cable bar half-kneeling chop	1-2	8 each side	Slow	60 sec
Resistance training			**SETS**	**REPS**	**TEMPO**	**REST**
	2.	Front squat	2-3	6	—	2 min+
	3a.	Chin-up	2-3	6	Mod	60 sec
	3b.	One-dumbbell block single-leg deadlift	2-3	6 each side	—	60 sec
	4a.	Barbell overhead press	2-3	6	Mod	60 sec
	4b.	Rope split-stance neutral-grip face pull with external rotation	2	10-12	Mod	60 sec

Table 6.8   Beginner to Intermediate Strength-Building Program: Phase 2, Day B

Core training			SETS	REPS	TEMPO	REST
	1a.	Sandbag full-dead bug with alternate-leg reach	1-2	5 each side	FE	N/A
	1b.	Side plank	1-2	4-6 each side	5 sec	60 sec
Resistance training			**SETS**	**REPS**	**TEMPO**	**REST**
	2.	Deadlift	2-3	6	—	2 min +
	3a.	Bench press	2-3	6	Mod	60 sec
	3b.	Goblet rear-foot-elevated split squat	2-3	6 each side	—	60 sec
	4a.	Dumbbell three-point neutral-grip row	2-3	6-8 each side	Mod	60 sec
	4b.	Swiss ball supine hip extension leg curl	2	8-10	Slow	60 sec

Advanced Program

This program is designed to be used by clients with a primary goal of strength who scored 15 points or more on our training age rubric discussed in chapter 2. It should not be used by clients who scored less than 15 points.

The client will alternate between session A, session B, session C and session D on each training day, performing each session at least four times in each phase (this could be extended if the client is still making progress). Phases 1 and 2 are each designed to be done for four to six weeks depending on how frequently the client trains each week. This also provides some flexibility. If the client trains with a frequency of three times per week (see table 6.9), phases 1 and 2 will each be completed in six weeks. This microcycle covers a 10-day period versus the traditional 7-day week. If the client trains four times per week (see table 6.10), each phase will take four weeks to complete, as shown in the charts below. Although a client could train four days per week on this type of weekly split, our recommendation is to train three days per week. See tables 6.11 through 6.18 for the sample advanced strength-building program.

Table 6.9   Advanced Phase 1 and 2 Sample Weekly Schedule: Three Sessions per Week

	Mon	Tues	Wed	Thurs	Fri	Sat	Sun
Week 1	Session A		Session B		Session C		
Week 2	Session D		Session A		Session B		
Week 3	Session C		Session D		Session A		
Week 4	Session B		Session C		Session D		
Week 5	Session A		Session B		Session C		
Week 6	Session D						

Table 6.10   Advanced Phase 1 and 2 Sample Weekly Schedule: Four Sessions per Week

	Mon	Tues	Wed	Thurs	Fri	Sat	Sun
Week 1	Session A	Session B		Session C	Session D		
Week 2	Session A	Session B		Session C	Session D		
Week 3	Session A	Session B		Session C	Session D		
Week 4	Session A	Session B		Session C	Session D		

Table 6.11   Advanced Strength-Building Program: Phase 1, Day A

Core training			SETS	REPS	TEMPO	REST
	1.	Suspension trainer kneeling fallout	2-3	6-8	Slow	60 sec
Resistance training			SETS	REPS	TEMPO	REST
	2a.	Back squat	3-4	5	—	90 sec
	2b.	Chin-up	3-4	4-7	Mod	90 sec
	3a.	Dumbbell two-point single-leg neutral-grip row	2-3	12 each side	—	60 sec
	3b.	Goblet cross-behind lunge	2-3	10 each side	—	60 sec

Table 6.12   Advanced Strength-Building Program: Phase 1, Day B

Core training			SETS	REPS	TEMPO	REST
	1.	Kettlebell single-arm waiter's walk	2-3	20 yd each direction	—	45 sec
Resistance training			SETS	REPS	TEMPO	REST
	2a.	Two-dumbbell single-leg Romanian deadlift	3-4	6 each side	Mod	90 sec
	2b.	Bench press	3-4	5	—	90 sec
	3a.	Suspension trainer leg curl	2-3	10	Slow	60 sec
	3b.	Dumbbell low-incline alternating neutral-grip bench press	2-3	8-10 each side	—	60 sec

Table 6.13   Advanced Strength-Building Program: Phase 1, Day C

Core training			SETS	REPS	TEMPO	REST
	1.	Hollow isometric hold	2-3	1	15-20 sec	45 sec
Resistance training			SETS	REPS	TEMPO	REST
	2a.	Single-leg squat to box	3-4	6 each side	—	90 sec
	2b.	Barbell overhand-grip dead row	3-4	8	—	90 sec
	3a.	Goblet lateral squat	2	10 each side	—	60 sec
	3b.	Kneeling alternating neutral-grip pulldown from bottom	2	8-10 each side	Mod	60 sec

Table 6.14   Advanced Strength-Building Program: Phase 1, Day D

Core training			SETS	REPS	TEMPO	REST
	1.	Cable bar half-kneeling chop	2-3	8 each side	Slow	45 sec
Resistance training			SETS	REPS	TEMPO	REST
	2a.	Deadlift	3-4	5	—	90 sec
	2b.	Barbell overhead press	3-4	5	Mod	90 sec
	3a.	Single-leg shoulder-elevated hip bridge	2-3	10-15 each side	Slow	60 sec
	3b.	Suspension trainer push-up	2	10-15	Mod	60 sec

Table 6.15   Advanced Strength-Building Program: Phase 2, Day A

Core training			SETS	REPS	TEMPO	REST
	1.	Wheel kneeling roll-out	2-3	5-7	Slow	60 sec
Resistance training			SETS	REPS	TEMPO	REST
	2a.	Back squat	3-4	3	—	90 sec
	2b.	Chin-up (ladder)*	3-4	1, 2, 3	Mod	90 sec
	3a.	Dumbbell three-point neutral-grip row	2-3	10 each side	Mod	60 sec
	3b.	Two-dumbbell cross-behind lunge	2-3	8 each side	—	60 sec

*This is a set and rep protocol that is popular within the StrongFirst community. One set equals one ladder, and each miniset of reps within each ladder (separated by a comma) equals one rung, then rest at least 30 to 60 seconds between rungs as needed. Start with approximately 5-6RM loads for the 1, 2, 3 ladders. If the prescribed reps are too challenging, don't start the "rung" (or miniset), and simply finish the rest of the ladders one rung lower. The top end rung should not be easy, but don't go to failure. For example, let's say the client did 2 sets of (1,2,3) and is shooting for 3 sets of (1,2,3). The client did a clean 3 reps on the first ladder and the next rung of 3 on the second ladder was hard. On the third ladder, the client finishes one rung lower, this means (1,2) not (1,2,2) This is one "rung" lower, not 1 rep lower. Finally, resistance can be increased once the prescribed rungs (mini sets of reps) and ladders (sets) have been completed.

Table 6.16   Advanced Strength-Building Program: Phase 2, Day B

Core training			SETS	REPS	TEMPO	REST
	1.	Kettlebell windmill	2-3	4-6 each side	Slow	60 sec
Resistance training			SETS	REPS	TEMPO	REST
	2a.	Barbell single-leg deadlift	3-4	4 each side	—	90 sec
	2b.	Bench press	3-4	3	—	90 sec
	3a.	Suspension trainer supine hip extension leg curl	2-3	8	Slow	60 sec
	3b.	Dip	2-3	6-8	Mod	60 sec

Table 6.17   Advanced Strength-Building Program: Phase 2, Day C

Core training			SETS	REPS	TEMPO	REST
	1.	Hollow rocking	2-3	15-20	—	45 sec
Resistance training			SETS	REPS	TEMPO	REST
	2a.	Single-leg squat from box	3-4	3 each side	—	90 sec
	2b.	Barbell overhand-grip dead row	3-4	6	—	90 sec
	3a.	One-dumbbell lateral lunge	2	8 each side	—	60 sec
	3b.	Suspension trainer overhand-grip inverted face pull with external rotation	2	6-8	Slow	60 sec

Table 6.18   Advanced Strength-Building Program: Phase 2, Day D

Core training			SETS	REPS	TEMPO	REST
	1.	Cable bar half-kneeling lift	2-3	8 each side	Slow	45 sec
Resistance training			SETS	REPS	TEMPO	REST
	2a.	Deadlift	3-4	3	—	90 sec
	2b.	Barbell overhead press	3-4	3	Mod	90 sec
	3a.	Single-leg shoulder-elevated hip bridge	2-3	8-12 each side	Slow	60 sec
	3b.	Suspension trainer push-up	2	8-12	Mod	60 sec

SELECT BEGINNER TO INTERMEDIATE STRENGTH-BUILDING PROGRAM EXERCISES

CABLE KNEELING UNDERHAND-GRIP PULLDOWN

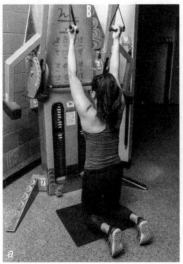 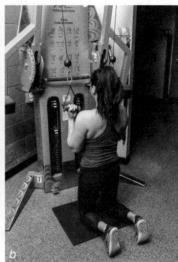

Setup and Performance

- Attach two handles to a high pulley on a functional trainer or a similar apparatus.
- Grasp the handles and get into a tall-kneeling posture with the palms turned toward the body.
- Leading with the shoulder blades, pull down so that the upper arms end at the sides of the torso.
- Return to the starting position and repeat.

Key Performance Points

- Keep the shoulders away from the ears in the bottom position.
- Brace the core and keep the ribs and hips together to maintain the core cylinder.
- We refer to the supinated grip as underhand grip to avoid confusion. This grip puts the biceps in a relatively leverage-advantaged position.

ONE-DUMBBELL STAGGERED-STANCE ROMANIAN DEADLIFT

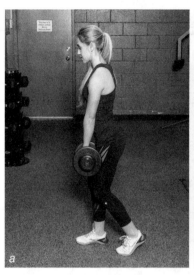 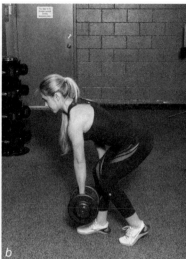

Setup and Performance

- Stand with feet hip-width apart and slide one foot back so the toe of the back foot is in line with the heel of the front foot, or up to a few inches behind it.
- Keep the back heel elevated off the floor, with most of the weight in the front foot. The back foot primarily serves as a kickstand.
- Hold one dumbbell in the hand of the back leg, opposite the front or working leg.
- With soft knees, push the hips back and bend forward, loading the hips. Push through the floor with the front foot and return to the starting position.

Key Performance Points

- Keep the spine stable. The movement comes through the hips, not the spine.
- Slide the shoulder blades down toward the back pockets and keep the shoulders square as the hip-hinging occurs.
- A posterior weight shift needs to occur to execute the movement properly; be sure the movement is coming from the hips and not from dropping the chest or arm down. The front shin should stay relatively vertical as if it is in a ski boot.
- Make sure the hips stay level without moving noticeably to the left or right. Keep the hips in the "center lane" as they go back.

BARBELL ROMANIAN DEADLIFT

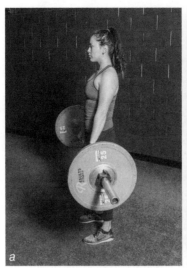 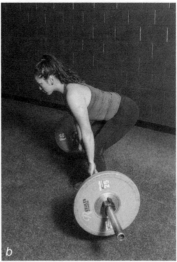

Setup and Performance

- Stand with the feet approximately hip-width apart with the hands slightly wider than shoulder-width apart, holding a barbell with an overhand grip.
- Grip the floor with the feet and perform a hip hinge by moving the hips backwards with a slight knee bend while bending forward. Keep the spine stable as the hips are moving backward.
- The bar will end somewhere between the bottom of the knees and midshin depending on one's build and mobility.
- When the hips can't move back any further, reverse the action and return to the starting position. Repeat.

Key Performance Points

- Keep the bar close the body at all times.
- Keep the ribs down and "hidden" slightly to prevent excessive lumbar hyperextension.
- Keep the neck in a relatively neutral position.

SUSPENSION TRAINER FRONT PLANK

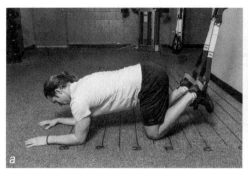 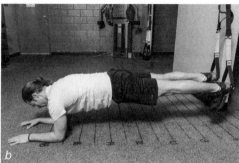

Setup and Performance

- Adjust the bottom of the foot straps so that they hang at midshin.
- Place the feet in the straps so that they are even when you are facing the ground.
- Get into a front plank position with the elbows stacked directly under the shoulder joints and the forearms parallel to each other.
- Hold the static plank position for the designated time.

Key Performance Points

- Keep the face pushed away from the ground and the neck in a neutral position.
- Keep the body long. If you are 5-foot 10-inches (178 cm) tall, make yourself 6-foot (183 cm) tall.
- Do not hyperextend the lumbar spine. Keep the buttons and belt buckle (the ribs and hips) together to maintain the core cylinder.
- Bring the knees under the hips at end of the set rather than just dropping the hips straight down once the rep is complete.

BARBELL OVERHEAD PRESS

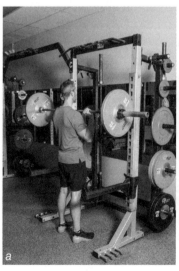 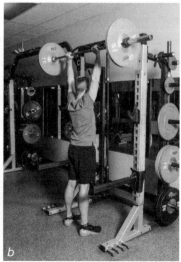

Setup and Performance

- Set a barbell in the rack uprights at about midchest level.
- Take the bar out of the rack using a shoulder-width grip so that the forearms are relatively vertical when viewed from the front and back, and the toes are turned slightly out.
- Keep the legs straight and extended in order to have a stable platform.
- Drive the bar overhead until the arms are straight and the upper arms are vertical with the bar line up over the middle of the foot.
- Lower the barbell with control to the starting position. Reset and repeat.

Key Performance Points

- The bar will be just below the collarbones at the starting position. Be sure not to take too wide nor too narrow a grip.
- Hold the bar deep in the hand near the palm, not the fingers.
- Keep the elbows slightly forward of the bar (as viewed from the side) when the bar is in the starting position.
- Press the bar close the face. The bar path should be in as straight a line as possible.

GOBLET REAR-FOOT-ELEVATED SPLIT SQUAT

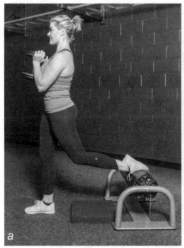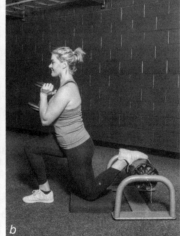

Setup and Performance

- Start by standing in a split stance holding one dumbbell or kettlebell in the goblet position in front of the chest.
- Elevate the rear leg on a circular split-squat stand or a flat exercise bench (a maximum height of about 16 to 18 inches [41-46 cm] works well for most people) with the laces down (the ankle plantar flexed).
- Bend the knees and lower the hips toward the floor. Drop relatively straight down.
- Push through the front foot and return to the top. Repeat.

Key Performance Points

- Ensure that the back knee, hip, and shoulder are relatively stacked or lined up at the bottom position of each split squat.
- The trailing leg's knee should not bang on the floor, it should almost touch the floor.
- The knee of the front leg will be stacked directly over the ankle as viewed from the front; it should not cave in.

ADVANCED STRENGTH-BUILDING PROGRAM EXERCISES

GOBLET CROSS-BEHIND LUNGE

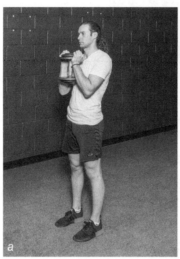 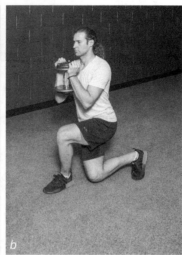

Setup and Performance

- Stand in a split stance holding one dumbbell or kettlebell in the goblet position in front of the chest with the feet about hip-width apart.
- Step back with one leg diagonally behind the front leg.
- Sit back and down so that the rear knee almost touches the ground.
- Push through the front foot and return to the starting position. Repeat.

Key Performance Points

- Keep the hips squared to the front.
- Before loading this movement, make sure to step the correct distance back and across by checking if the knee of the back leg drops to the outside and just behind of the heel of the stationary leg.

KETTLEBELL SINGLE-ARM WAITER'S WALK

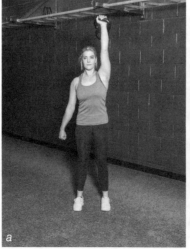 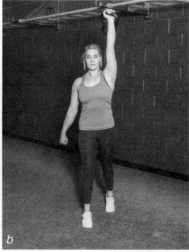

Setup and Performance

- Hold a kettlebell in the rack position and press it overhead.
- The kettlebell will sit on the forearm; keep the wrist neutral and straight.
- Keeping the arm vertical, walk the required distance and then switch arms.

Key Performance Points

- Keep the torso vertical.
- Cue the client to keep the "shoulder out of the ear" to create tension and stability.
- Keep the elbow straight.
- Keep the opposite arm relatively close to the side to prevent it from becoming a counter-weight.

SUSPENSION TRAINER LEG CURL

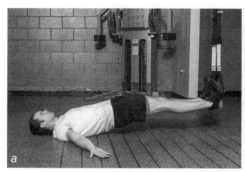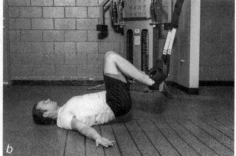

Setup and Performance

- Adjust the bottom of the foot straps so that they hang at midshin.
- Place the heels in the foot straps and lay supine on the back with the palms up.
- Set the core and lift up the hips so that the body forms a straight line from the shoulders, hips, and knees.
- Pull the heels toward the butt while keeping the hips in place and the core braced. The hips and knees will flex together in the leg curl.
- Push the heels away and repeat, keeping the hips in the same position for the entire set.

Key Performance Points

- The pelvis should stay stationary throughout the whole exercise. It should not move up or down while the knees and hip flex and extend.
- At the finish position, the thighs should be vertical.

HOLLOW ISOMETRIC HOLD

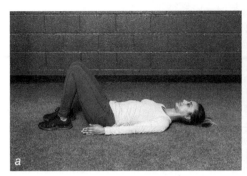
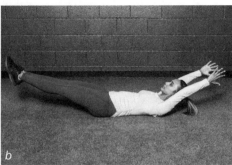

Setup and Performance

- Start by lying on the back with the knees bent.
- Pull the bottom of the ribs toward the top of the pelvis. Press the lower back slightly into the floor.
- Lift the legs off the floor and extend the arms overhead.
- Keep the legs straight and the toes pointed. The body will be in a slight curve, resembling a banana shape.
- Hold for the designated time in this position taking short, hissing breaths.

Key Performance Points

- The hollow position and name comes to us from gymnastics. It's not the old idea of sucking in the abs. It is locking the rib cage down to the pelvis and keeping that distance when forces are trying to pull it apart.
- The key is to create tension from the tips of the toes through the fingertips.
- Maintain the distance between the rib cage and pelvis. They must stayed "tied" together as you hold.

BARBELL OVERHAND-GRIP DEAD ROWS

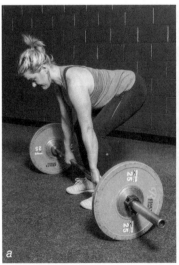
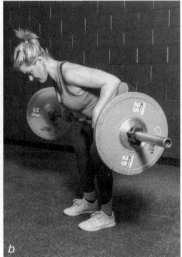

Setup and Performance

- Stand with the feet shoulder-width apart in front of a loaded barbell. Bend over and grab the bar with a shoulder-width grip or slightly wider.
- Bend the knees while keeping the hips high and the back flat. Take a big deep breath, brace against the weight, and pull it toward the bottom of the sternum or abdominal line.
- Return the weight back to the ground, reset, and repeat. Every repetition will start from a complete dead stop with the bar on the floor as in a true deadlift.

Key Performance Points

- Don't round the back. Keep a neutral back and neck position throughout the exercise.
- Take up the slack before picking up the bar rather than jerking the bar off the floor.
- If the torso rises too far above horizontal, the weight is too heavy.
- The resetting of the bar on the floor after each rep staves off excessive fatigue of the low-back musculature since it is not held in a continuous isometric action like most versions of the barbell row.

SINGLE-LEG SHOULDER-ELEVATED HIP BRIDGE

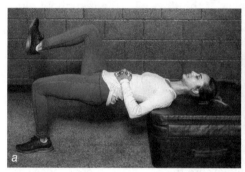 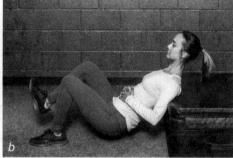

Setup and Performance

- Use a sturdy bench or padded box that is about 12 to 16 inches (30-41 cm) high. Facing up, place the bottom of the shoulder blades on the edge of the box.
- Start with both feet flat and a 90-degree bend in the knee with both hips bridged up to the top position.
- Remove one foot off the floor and flex the hip and knee to 90-degrees.
- Lower the hips straight down and then return under control to the top position. Repeat.

Key Performance Points

- Brace the core and keep the ribs and hips together to maintain the core cylinder. It is common to try to substitute lumbar hyperextension for hip extension in this exercise.
- Keep the neck neutral and in line with the spine; there is a tendency to hyperextend the neck when the hips are lowered.
- The shoulders should not slide on the box; they are a pivot point.

TWO-DUMBBELL CROSS-BEHIND LUNGE

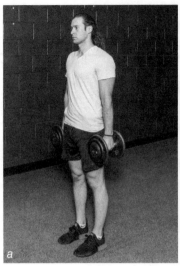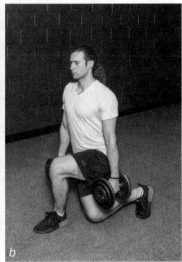

Setup and Performance

- Stand in a split stance holding two dumbbells at the sides with the feet about hip-width apart.
- Step back with one leg diagonally behind the front leg.
- Sit back and down so that the rear knee almost touches the ground.
- Push through the front foot and return to the starting position. Repeat.

Key Performance Points

- Keep the hips squared to the front.
- Before loading this movement, make sure make sure to step the correct distance back and across by checking if the knee of the back leg drops to the outside and just behind of the heel of the stationary leg.

KETTLEBELL WINDMILL

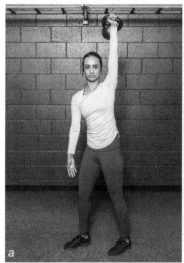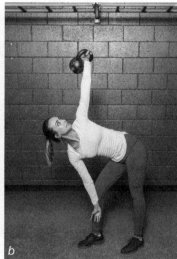

Setup and Performance

- Hold a kettlebell in one hand and press it overhead. Set the feet to about shoulder-width apart.
- Turn both feet out at about a 45-degree angle away from the side that is holding the kettlebell (or toward the side that is not holding the kettlebell).
- The leg that is in back (the side of the kettlebell) will stay straight. Shift the weight into the back leg and put a slight bend in the knee of the front leg. Keep the arm holding the kettlebell vertical at all times.
- Perform a diagonal hip-hinge and rotate through the upper back until the back arm holding the kettlebell is now turned up toward the ceiling creating a T with the arms.
- Return to the top and repeat.

Key Performance Points

- The weight distribution should be about 70 percent on the back leg and 30 percent on the front leg.
- The free arm can reach for the ground (although touching the ground is not the goal), or it can provide a guide by gliding down the front of the leg.
- Go down only as far as mobility allows.

BARBELL SINGLE-LEG DEADLIFT

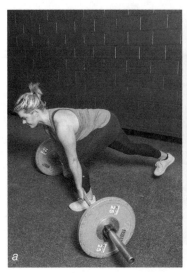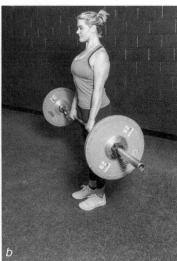

Setup and Performance

- Set up a loaded barbell on the floor as if to perform a conventional deadlift but put both feet together instead of hip-width apart. You will hold the bar with an overhand grip that is about shoulder-width apart (arms and hand straight down).
- Pick up one foot and extend it behind the body, straightening the knee.
- The hips will be higher than the knees but lower than the shoulder in the starting position.
- Create tension and "push" the slack out of the bar before attempting to lift the bar.
- Push the floor away and move to a fully standing position, keeping the bar close to the body at all times.
- Return the bar to the floor in the reverse manner. Reset the bar on the floor fully (i.e., the floor will take the weight of the bar) and repeat.

Key Performance Points

- Recall that a true deadlift starts with "dead" weight on the floor or on a block at the start of each rep.
- Keep the back leg extended and relatively low to the ground. A common mistake is to try to lift the leg too high toward the ceiling on the lowering portion of the lift.
- Keep the stance or working leg bent at the bottom of the movement; this is critical as it allows the hips to move back properly, if the hips don't move back, they may spin open and balance will be compromised.
- Keep the spine stable and in a relatively straight line (not to confused with vertical) during the movement.

SUSPENSION TRAINER OVERHAND-GRIP INVERTED FACE PULL WITH EXTERNAL ROTATION

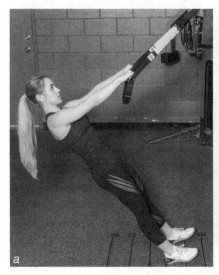 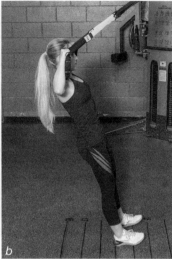

Setup and Performance

- Set the suspension trainer handles in the fully shortened position to about the top of hip height. Keeping the arms straight and holding on to the handles, walk the feet down to create the proper body angle for an appropriately challenging set of repetitions.
- Holding on to the straps with the palms facing down in an overhand grip, keep the heels planted into ground with the toes pulled forward, and find a strong plank position.
- Pull the body toward the anchor point with the elbows up and rotating the handles toward the forehead. Lower the body back down, maintaining the plank position, and repeat.

Key Performance Points

- Keep the eyes focused on the anchor point (where the suspension trainer is attached) to help maintain a neutral head and neck position throughout the movement.
- Maintain one smooth motion throughout the pull.
- Brace the core and keep the ribs and hips together to maintain the core cylinder during the execution of this movement.

CABLE BAR HALF-KNEELING LIFT

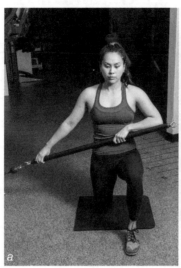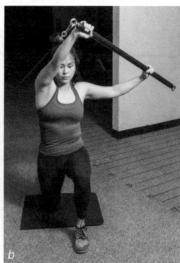

Setup and Performance

- Attach a cable bar or a long rope to an adjustable cable machine to a low pulley. Get into a half-kneeling position next to the machine and turn perpendicular to the pulley.
- The outside knee (the leg furthest from the weight stack) should be up. Use an overhand grip.
- Pull the bar across the body keeping the bar close to the torso, and then press both arms out at the top moving the cable in a diagonal line.
- The bar moves in a low to high manner.

Key Performance Points

- Be sure to keep the torso stacked through the whole movement. Keep the rib cage stacked over the hips. Think of this as a half-kneeling plank.
- There will be some rotation and motion through the upper back and shoulders but keep the hips static.

CHAPTER 7

General Fitness Programs

People come to see you for one of three primary reasons:

1. They want to look better (lose fat or gain muscle).
2. They want to perform better in a physical pursuit or sporting activity.
3. They want to improve how they feel and move.

We have addressed the first two reasons in previous chapters, and this chapter will address the third reason. As legendary strength coach Mike Boyle has said, "People will continue to pay you if you make them feel better." This is a simple statement, but it is very true. Not everyone that comes to see you will be looking to push the limits in terms of physique or physical performance. Some just want to move and feel better to improve their overall quality of life over the short and long term, do something they perceive is good for them, and reduce life stress.

Most people know that they should exercise for a host of beneficial reasons. Certainly, one of the most results-producing forms of exercise for an aging population is resistance training, because it combats some of the effects of aging. In particular, we know that it improves bone density and staves off muscle and power loss. Generally, good sensible training practices will make people feel better overall. The adept fitness professional can literally change someone's life by providing this service.

People who are looking for these more general, nonspecific, or hard-to-measure-type goals would be classified as general fitness clients. They want a little bit of everything, but not too much of one thing. Most of the time, this demographic will be females and males in the age bracket of 40 years old and up, and will often have a very low training age when starting out. It's often difficult to pin them down to any specific goals (though we always work to do so). Their goals (such as they are) can be hard to measure because they tend to be quite subjective.

Also, for many of these clients, working out or training is often very hard for them. In other words, just getting to the gym two to three times per week is quite an accomplishment, so we can't lose sight of their personal experiences since we are all at different points along our training journey. The accomplishment of an actual training session is often secondary to the triumph of making it through the door and establishing the habit of training on a regular basis. Once these routines are established, you never know what direction training will take. What often begins as general fitness can evolve into something entirely new once these routines and habits have been established. That's one of the reasons it is so important to have conversations about goals, and to discuss what clients want from their training on a regular basis as part of your coaching and program system. We discuss how to implement this in our system in chapter 10.

Some of our general fitness clients often have a hard time being comfortable with getting uncomfortable early on in their training journeys. This concept can be difficult for fitness coaches to appreciate because exercising is our "easy." In fact, this "easy" is often one of the reasons we get into this industry in the first place. As such, it's often difficult for coaches to have empathy for those whom exercise doesn't come easy. Think about something that is hard for you. Maybe it's managing your personal finances, or maybe it's being organized. For others, this comes very easily, but for you it is really challenging. Exercising can be the same way for someone else. If you are going to get buy-in from your clients, you must put yourself in their shoes and see things from their perspective. This is why communication and asking the right open-ended questions from the outset is so critical in understanding what these types of clients are requesting from you. The fine folks at Precision Nutrition have taught us that each of us has our own different "hard" and "easy." If you think about it in this manner, you will be able to help your clients build better behavior habits and set them up for success. Empathy is the basis for all of our meaningful relationships, and is fundamental to building trust with clients; it must be earned by truly caring and being able to demonstrate that you care.

One great way to show that you care is to find out how your clients are doing by regularly asking questions. Two simple questions to ask on regular basis to help build connection and a meaningful relationship (that we learned from our colleague Tristan Rice of EXOS) are: (1) Do you feel better than when you got here? and (2) Do you feel like you have made progress toward your goals today?

Now that we provided some background context, let's get into the practical aspects of how to do this in the real world.

Programming Without a Specific Goal

Programming for this population can be somewhat challenging because of the lack of a clear and specific goal. It can be very subjective to measure results because a lot is based on how the client feels. This is compounded by the fact that this population has a lot of variation and diversity of personality types. It is challenging for sure.

It is often hard to nail down specifics and fit these clients into our SMART (specific, measurable, attainable, relevant, and time-based) goal framework discussed in chapter 1. We have to take some liberties and train for multiple qualities with a generalist approach to be able to create some general training objectives for these clients.

Increase Strength on Basic Foundational Exercises

Using primarily resistance training, we are going to train the client to get stronger for a given number of reps. When choosing a quality to emphasize, we typically favor a strength-based approach because of the "rope ladder" phenomenon and the return on investment discussed in chapter 6. Foundational exercises that we focus on for this demographic will include the following:

- Goblet squat
- Kettlebell or hex bar deadlift
- Suspension trainer inverted row or chin-up
- Dumbbell row
- Push-up
- Kettlebell single-arm overhead press

- Split squat
- Dumbbell or Kettlebell single-leg deadlift
- Plank variation and chop and lift variation

With general population clients we typically do most of our work in the 6 to 15 rep range, which is the traditional hypertrophy rep range. Why do we use this range if the goal is strength? We use it because loads above 85 percent of 1RM carry a bit more risk. When we are trying to improve the general quality of strength, we still achieve neurological strength gains in the 6 to 10 rep range (just not as much as with heavier loads). As discussed in chapter 6, there are several definitions of strength, with only one that involves 1RM absolute maximum. Remember that getting stronger in any rep range is still getting stronger.

Include Appropriate Amount of Variety

When most people hear the word *variety*, they often think in terms of exercises. This is certainly one way to provide variety, but as you have previously seen, we primarily implement it through varying repetitions. Because the training goals are much more general, there is typically more room for exercise variety in the training of general fitness clients. Without a doubt, we still want to develop competency and proficiency

---

What's Strong Enough for General Fitness Folks?

The first question to ask the general fitness client is, "How strong do you need to be?" That's a really hard question to answer and it is obviously dependent on each individual, but we can provide some general thoughts. We feel that at a minimum, these clients need the strength to be resilient in the game of life and to handle the stresses that they encounter in activities of daily living (ADL) with a bit of an extra buffer or reserve. Some general fitness clients need to be even stronger for recreational sporting pursuits, but at that point they are actually starting to spill over into a different client category so their needs and programming will change.

We have seen far too many clients using weight for deadlifts that is lighter than a bag of groceries that they routinely pick up. Their purses and backpacks often weigh more than the kettlebell they just deadlifted for 10 reps. We are not saying that everyone needs to be deadlifting 400 pounds (181 kg), but we need to be conscious about providing an appropriate training stress to achieve adaptations. When there is fear or apprehension about lifting certain loads in the gym, it is often helpful to frame it with examples such as the grocery bag or purse to give clients perspective and confidence that they can do this. We often have to have some delicate conversations about effort levels. We have to show them that we believe in them more than they believe in themselves.

We will push and nudge them to succeed at these basic exercises, and progress from there as warranted. Once we achieve some benchmarks, progression won't always come in the form of increased load, but often in the form of intensiveness by making an exercise feel harder via tempo changes, off-set loading with odd implements, and other exercise variety. In this manner we can increase challenge and stress without the excessive risk of pushing load too often with an aging population. Risk versus reward must always be taken into account.

in the basic fundamental movements, but once we do, we can layer in some exercise variety. As a guideline, the lower the training age, the less variety that is required.

Exercise variety is often a double-edged sword. With general fitness clients it either happens way too often or not at all. In our experience, most newer coaches have a tendency to get too sexy too soon. The biggest trap that many newer coaches can fall into is what we first heard Mark Verstegen call "enter-trainment." This is, quite simply, random variety for the sake of keeping a client engaged with newness and shiny objects. Whenever you are going to vary something in a program, you must have a purpose and it should not be selected for the coolness and sexiness factor. That is simply randomness, which does not produce results.

Some reasons to include more exercise variety in the programming for general fitness clients would be the following:

- *Provide movement variability and diverse movement experiences.* Life and sport occur in all three planes of motion; therefore, our training must prepare us to do so. We want to balance a degree of baseline strength along with training outside the sagittal plane of motion.
- *Alleviate boredom with an exercise.* Eating chicken and broccoli everyday would get old after some time; likewise, we all need a break from the monotony of doing the same exercise over and over. Too often clients say they are bored with an exercise after one or two sessions. That's silly. But if they mention that they are sick of an exercise after performing it for a reasonable amount of time, then you should consider changing it. If the client feels like they are making a death-march to the gym because they *have* to do an exercise, that's not good. We discussed the trap of "enter-trainment," but keep in mind that you don't want to go too far in the opposite direction. Training needs to be somewhat enjoyable, and there are some sensible spices that we throw into our training programs from time to time without compromising the effectiveness.

Standards for General Fitness Populations

It can be helpful to use some attainable minimum strength standards for this population. This helps the fitness professional provide some purpose to the training of general fitness clients and guide them to what they need. We talked about strength in the previous chapter, and we can apply it on a different scale with this population. Stronger is almost always going to be better, and it's the physical quality that we can most directly impact with these clients.

Table 7.1 provides a handful of exercise standards that we steer most of our general fitness clients toward to ensure that their strength is at a very minimum. These are starting points of the journey. They also serve as benchmarks of progress to different exercise progressions for other client demographics. They are guidelines only and must be viewed as such.

General Fitness Programming

In terms of periodization for our rep programming, we use a nonlinear alternating periodization rep scheme (see table 1.2 in chapter 1 for an overview) for both the beginner to intermediate phases and for the advanced phases. This type of periodization scheme tends to work well over the long term because we alternate each mesocycle between higher reps to accumulate volume and relatively lower reps in the following

Table 7.1   General Fitness Standards

Movement pattern	Exercise	Females	Males
Pull	Inverted row	5 reps with vertical straps set at hip height	5 reps with vertical straps set at hip height
Squat (symmetrical stance)	Goblet squat	0.5 × BW, 10 reps (or too heavy to hold in position)	0.5 × BW, 10 reps (or too heavy to hold in position)
Hip hinge (symmetrical stance)	Kettlebell deadlift	48 kg (106 lb), 10 reps	48 kg (106 lb), 10 reps
	High hex bar deadlift	1.0 × BW, 6 reps	1.0 × BW, 6 reps
Push	Push-up	5 reps +	10 reps +
Hip hinge (single-leg)	One-kettlebell single-leg Romanian deadlift	16 kg (35 lb), 8 reps each side	24 kg (53 lb), 8 reps each side
Squat (split stance)	Two-dumbbell split squat	20 lb (9 kg) each dumb-bell, 8 reps each side	30 lb (14 kg) each dumb-bell, 8 reps each side
	Goblet rear-foot-elevated split squat	30 lb (14 kg), 8 reps each side	45-50 lb (20-23 kg), 8 reps each side
Core	Front plank	60 sec	60 sec
	Side plank	30 sec each side	30 sec each side

mesocycle to build more strength. The late Charles Poliquin was probably the first to popularize this approach and following is our application of this concept.

In terms of a weekly split, an A and B session full-body split works really well for general fitness clients regardless of training age. They tend to train two to three times per week, so it works far better than having a fixed day schedule or an upper and lower split.

Let's now delve into the specifics and see what programming for our general fitness actually looks like in practice.

Beginner to Intermediate Program

As in previous chapters, this program is designed to be used by clients who scored below 15 on our training age rubric discussed in chapter 2. Apply the same exercise progression and regression principles to these selected exercises to ensure that they are a fit for your client.

The client will alternate between session A and session B on each training day, performing session A six times and session B six times in each phase. Phases 1 and 2 are each designed to be done for four to six weeks, depending on how frequently the client trains each week. This also provides some flexibility. If the client trains with a frequency of three times per week, which is optimal (see table 7.2), phases 1 and 2 will each be completed in four weeks, and if training two times per week (see table

Table 7.2   Beginner to Intermediate Phase 1 and 2 Sample Weekly Schedule: Three Sessions per Week

	Mon	Tues	Wed	Thurs	Fri	Sat	Sun
Week 1	Session A		Session B		Session A		
Week 2	Session B		Session A		Session B		
Week 3	Session A		Session B		Session A		
Week 4	Session B		Session A		Session B		

7.3), it will take six weeks to complete each phase. After completing all of the A and B sessions for phase 1, the client moves on to phase 2. See tables 7.4 through 7.7 for the sample beginner to intermediate general fitness program (the tempo key is on page 29).

Table 7.3   Beginner to Intermediate Phase 1 and 2 Sample Weekly Schedule: Two Sessions per Week

	Mon	Tues	Wed	Thurs	Fri	Sat	Sun
Week 1	Session A			Session B			
Week 2	Session A			Session B			
Week 3	Session A			Session B			
Week 4	Session A			Session B			
Week 5	Session A			Session B			
Week 6	Session A			Session B			

Table 7.4   Beginner to Intermediate General Fitness Program: Phase 1, Day A

Core training			SETS	REPS	TEMPO	REST
	1a.	Front plank	1-2	1	30-45 sec	0 sec
	1b.	Cable tall-kneeling antirotation press	1-2	10 each side	1-3-1	60 sec
Combination or power development			SETS	REPS	TEMPO	REST
	2.	Medicine ball tall-kneeling forward push throw	3-4	5	X	30 sec
Resistance training			SETS	REPS	TEMPO	REST
	3a.	Goblet squat	1-2	12	—	60 sec
	3b.	Cable half-kneeling single-arm neutral-grip row	1-2	10-12 each side	—	60 sec
	4a.	One-dumbbell staggered-stance Romanian deadlift	1-2	12 each side	—	60 sec
	4b.	Push-up	1-2	12	—	60 sec

Table 7.5   Beginner to Intermediate General Fitness Program: Phase 1, Day B

Core training			SETS	REPS	TEMPO	REST
	1a.	Sandbag dead bug with alternate-leg reach	1-2	5 each side	FE	0 sec
	1b.	Side plank from knees	1-2	4-6 each side	5 sec	60 sec
Combination or power development			SETS	REPS	TEMPO	REST
	2.	Medicine ball slam	3-4	5	X	30 sec
Resistance training			SETS	REPS	TEMPO	REST
	3a.	Kettlebell deadlift	1-2	12	—	60 sec
	3b.	Fulcrum half-kneeling single-arm press	1-2	10-12 each side	—	60 sec
	4a.	Goblet split squat	1-2	12 each side	—	60 sec
	4b.	Kneeling neutral-grip pulldown	1-2	10-12	—	60 sec

Table 7.6 Beginner to Intermediate General Fitness Program: Phase 2, Day A

Core training			SETS	REPS	TEMPO	REST
	1a.	Suspension trainer front plank	1-2	1	30-45 sec	0 sec
	1b.	Cable bar half-kneeling chop	1-2	8 each side	Slow	60 sec
Combination or power development			SETS	REPS	TEMPO	REST
	2.	Medicine ball standing forward push throw	3-4	5	X	30 sec
Resistance training			SETS	REPS	TEMPO	REST
	3a.	One-dumbbell single-leg Romanian deadlift	2-3	10 each side	—	60 sec
	3b.	Push-up	2-3	8-10	—	60 sec
	4a.	Goblet squat	2-3	8-10	—	60 sec
	4b.	Cable split-stance single-arm neutral-grip row	2-3	8-10 each side	—	60 sec

Table 7.7 Beginner to Intermediate General Fitness Program: Phase 2, Day B

Core training			SETS	REPS	TEMPO	REST
	1a.	Sandbag full-dead bug with alternate reach	1-2	5 each side	FE	0 sec
	1b.	Side plank	1-2	4-6 each side	5 sec	60 sec
Combination or power development			SETS	REPS	TEMPO	REST
	2.	Medicine ball side-rotational scoop throw	2-3	5 each side	X	20 sec
Resistance training			SETS	REPS	TEMPO	REST
	3a.	Two-dumbbell split squat	2-3	10 each side	—	60 sec
	3b.	Suspension trainer inverted neutral-grip row	2-3	8-10	Mod	60 sec
	4a.	High hex bar deadlift	2-3	10	—	60 sec
	4b.	Kettlebell half-kneeling single-arm overhead press	2-3	8-10 each side	—	60 sec

Advanced Program

This program is designed to be used by general fitness clients who scored 15 points or more on our training age rubric discussed in chapter 2. It should not be used by clients who scored less than 15 points.

The client will alternate between session A and session B on each training day, performing session A six times and session B six times in each phase. Phases 1 and 2 are each designed to be done for four to six weeks depending on how frequently the client trains each week. This also provides some flexibility. If the client trains with a frequency of three times per week (see table 7.8), phases 1 and 2 will be completed in four weeks, and if training two times per week (see table 7.9), it will take six weeks to complete each phase. See tables 7.10 through 7.13 for the sample advanced general fitness program.

Table 7.8 Advanced Phase 1 and 2 Sample Weekly Schedule: Three Sessions per Week

	Mon	Tues	Wed	Thurs	Fri	Sat	Sun
Week 1	Session A		Session B		Session A		
Week 2	Session B		Session A		Session B		
Week 3	Session A		Session B		Session A		
Week 4	Session B		Session A		Session B		

Table 7.9 Advanced Phase 1 and 2 Sample Weekly Schedule: Two Sessions per Week

	Mon	Tues	Wed	Thurs	Fri	Sat	Sun
Week 1	Session A			Session B			
Week 2	Session A			Session B			
Week 3	Session A			Session B			
Week 4	Session A			Session B			
Week 5	Session A			Session B			
Week 6	Session A			Session B			

Table 7.10 Advanced General Fitness Program: Phase 1, Day A

Core training			SETS	REPS	TEMPO	REST
	1.	Sandbag tall-plank lateral isometric hold (alternating)	2	4 each side	3 sec	60 sec
Combination or power development			SETS	REPS	TEMPO	REST
	2.	Kettlebell swing	3-4	10	X	45 sec
Resistance training			SETS	REPS	TEMPO	REST
	3a.	Goblet squat with 3 sec pause	2-3	10	2-3-0	60 sec
	3b.	Suspension trainer under-hand-grip inverted row	2-3	8-10	Mod	60 sec
	4a.	Single-leg shoulder-elevated hip bridge	2-3	8-10 each side	—	60 sec
	4b.	Dumbbell alternating neutral-grip bench press	2-3	8-10 each side	—	60 sec

Table 7.11 Advanced General Fitness Program: Phase 1, Day B

Core training			SETS	REPS	TEMPO	REST
	1.	Kettlebell single-arm bottoms-up rack walk	2	20 yd each direction	—	60 sec
Combination or power development			SETS	REPS	TEMPO	REST
	2.	Medicine ball side-rotational throw with step	3-4	5 each side	X	30 sec
Resistance training			SETS	REPS	TEMPO	REST
	3a.	High hex bar deadlift	2-3	10	—	60 sec
	3b.	Spiderman push-up (alternating)	2-3	5 each side	—	60 sec
	4a.	Single-leg skater squat	2-3	10 each side	—	60 sec
	4b.	Cable split-stance single-arm neutral-grip low row	2-3	8-10 each side	—	60 sec

Table 7.12 Advanced General Fitness Program: Phase 2, Day A

Core training			SETS	REPS	TEMPO	REST
	1.	Kettlebell single-arm waiter's walk	2	20 yd each direction	—	60 sec
Combination or power development			SETS	REPS	TEMPO	REST
	2.	Medicine ball cross-behind rotational side-scoop throw	3-4	4 each side	X	20 sec
Resistance training			SETS	REPS	TEMPO	REST
	3a.	One-dumbbell single-leg Romanian deadlift (contra)	2-3	6 each side	2-1-1	60 sec
	3b.	Dumbbell incline single-arm bench press	2-3	5-7 each side	Mod	60 sec
	4a.	Goblet one-and-a-half squat	2-3	6	—	60 sec
	4b.	One-dumbbell hand-supported single-leg neutral-grip row	2-3	6 each side	—	60 sec

Table 7.13 Advanced General Fitness Program: Phase 2, Day B

Core training			SETS	REPS	TEMPO	REST
	1.	Sandbag tall-plank lateral drag	2	4 each direction	—	60 sec
Combination or power development			SETS	REPS	TEMPO	REST
	2.	Kettlebell side-step swing	2-3	4 each side	X	45 sec
Resistance training			SETS	REPS	TEMPO	REST
	3a.	Single-leg squat to box	2-3	6 each side	—	60 sec
	3b.	Eccentric-only chin-up	2-3	3-5	4-6 sec	60 sec
	4a.	Slider eccentric-only supine hip extension leg curl	2-3	6-8	3 sec	60 sec
	4b.	Suspension trainer feet-suspended push-up	2-3	6-8	Mod	60 sec

SELECT BEGINNER TO INTERMEDIATE GENERAL FITNESS PROGRAM EXERCISES

MEDICINE BALL TALL-KNEELING FORWARD PUSH THROW

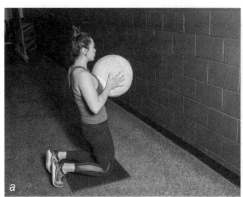 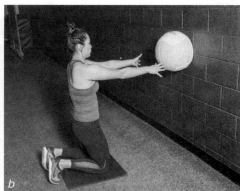

Setup and Performance

- Start in a tall-kneeling position about one-and-a-half arms distance from a solid brick wall.
- Push the ball into the wall as hard and fast as possible. Reset and repeat.

Key Performance Points

- Sound is a great tool for feedback. The louder the throw is the harder you threw it.
- Brace the core and keep the ribs and hips together to maintain the core cylinder.
- Maintain the tall-kneeling position while throwing the ball.

CABLE HALF-KNEELING SINGLE-ARM NEUTRAL-GRIP ROW

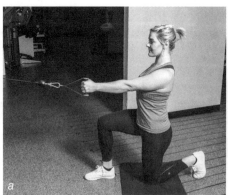 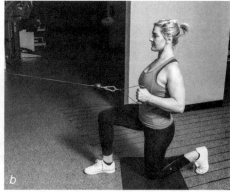

Setup and Performance

- Set a pulley to about waist height when standing. Grab the handle with the palm facing the body (the handle will be vertical) and get into a half-kneeling position facing the weight stack.
- Hold the handle opposite the leg that is up (e.g., if the left knee is up, hold the handle with the right hand).
- Pull the handle back by the side of ribs and then return to the starting position. Repeat.

Key Performance Points

- Ensure that you are in a properly aligned half-kneeling position with the back knee, hip, and shoulder aligned and stacked.
- Initiate the pull with the shoulder blade rather than the elbow.
- Be sure that the shoulder blades move with the upper arm as opposed to only bending the elbow.
- Keep the torso vertical and stable.

FULCRUM HALF-KNEELING SINGLE-ARM PRESS

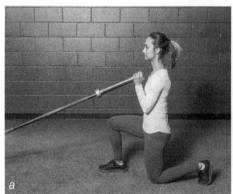 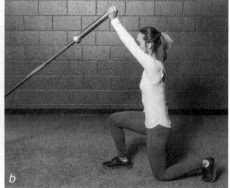

Setup and Performance

- Position a barbell in a "landmine" unit (we call this a *fulcrum* in our nomenclature) and then get into a half-kneeling position.
- Hold the end of the barbell on the down leg side.
- Press the weight up and away at an angle with a reach.
- With control, return to the starting position and repeat.

Key Performance Points

- Create cross body tension by making a tight fist in the opposite hand.
- Ensure that you are in a properly aligned half-kneeling position with the back knee, hip, and shoulder aligned and stacked.

ONE-DUMBBELL SINGLE-LEG ROMANIAN DEADLIFT

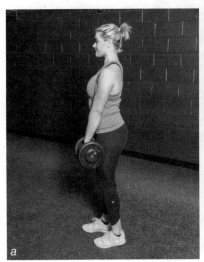 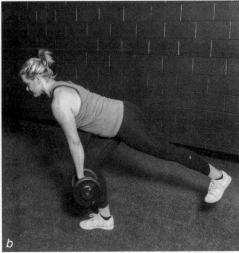

Setup and Performance

- Stand with both feet hip-width apart and then pick up one foot. The dumbbell will be on the same side as the leg that is going back.
- Hip-hinge on the working leg while the rear leg moves back. A straight line should be formed from the rear leg to the head.
- The dumbbell will be lowered in a straight line to a position that is somewhere between the level of the bottom of the knee and midshin.
- Push the floor away and hip-hinge to return to the start position while pulling the dumbbell up in a straight line. Repeat.

Key Performance Points

- In a Romanian deadlift the exercise starts with the weight at the top of the movement, and the weight will not go to the floor or a block to a "dead" weight position.
- Keep the spine stable, and move through the hips. Be sure to establish this position at the beginning, before the lift begins.
- Be sure to keep the working leg bent at the bottom of the movement. This is critical because it allows the hips to move back properly; if the hips don't move back, they will spin open and balance will be compromised.
- Keep the shoulders square at the bottom.

CABLE SPLIT-STANCE SINGLE-ARM NEUTRAL-GRIP ROW

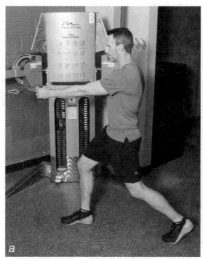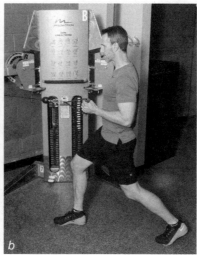

Setup and Performance

- Set a pulley to about midchest height when standing. Grab the handle with the palm facing the body (the handle will be vertical) and get into a split-stance (top of split squat) position facing the weight stack.
- Hold the handle opposite the leg that is up (e.g., if the left knee is up, hold the handle with the right hand).
- Pull the handle back by the side of the ribs and then return to the starting position. Repeat.

Key Performance Points

- Ensure that the hips are squared and the shoulders are aligned.
- Initiate the pull with the shoulder blade rather than the elbow.
- Be sure that the shoulder blades move with the upper arm as opposed to only bending the elbow.
- Keep the core braced and the torso vertical and stable.

MEDICINE BALL SIDE-ROTATIONAL SCOOP THROW

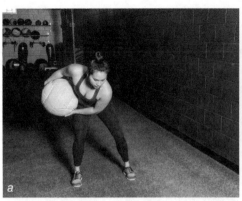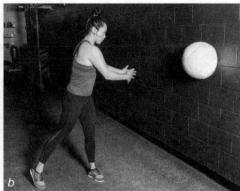

Setup and Performance

- Holding a medicine ball in the hands, turn sideways to the wall and about two arms distance from it.
- Set the feet a bit wider than shoulder-width apart with the hips pushed back, holding the ball with both hands across the body.
- Sit back and slightly down while turning the shoulders perpendicular to the hips.
- Strongly drive the floor away while rotating open and throw the ball into the wall explosively, turning the hips at the wall on the follow-through.
- Catch the ball, reset, and repeat.

Key Performance Points

- Throw the ball hard; try to break the ball.
- Sit into the hips to properly load them for the throw. The hips are the motor.
- Scoop the ball with both hands as it is thrown.

HIGH HEX BAR DEADLIFT

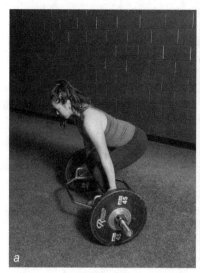 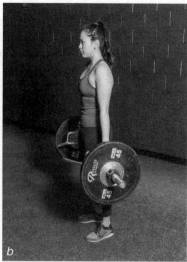

Setup and Performance

- Stand inside the frame of a loaded hex bar with the feet about hip-width apart or slightly narrower. Line up the middle of the bar with the middle of the foot.
- Bend over and grab the middle of the high handles and keep the arms straight.
- The hips will be higher than the knees but lower than the shoulders in the starting position.
- At the beginning of the movement, focus on a point about 7 to 10 feet ahead.
- Push the floor away and move to a fully standing position, moving the bar in a straight line.
- Return the bar to the floor in the reverse manner. Reset the bar on the floor fully (i.e., the floor will take the weight of the bar) and repeat.

Key Performance Points

- The deadlift is primarily a hip hinge, not a pure squat. The biggest mistake that most people make is setting the hips too low at the bottom of the movement.
- Create tension and "push" the slack out of the bar before attempting to actually lift the bar.

ADVANCED GENERAL FITNESS PROGRAM EXERCISES

SANDBAG TALL-PLANK LATERAL ISOMETRIC HOLD (ALTERNATING)

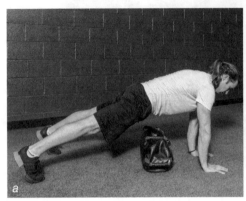 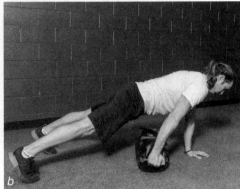

Setup and Performance

- Start in a typical push-up position with the hands under the shoulders and the legs straight.
- Set the feet wider than shoulder-width apart and position the bag directly underneath the body and slightly in front of the belly button.
- Pick up one hand while keeping the hips stable, and pull on the outside handle of the sandbag; take the slack out of the bag without actually moving the bag.
- Put the hand back on the floor and switch sides. Repeat.

Key Performance Points

- Maintain a stable pelvis while pulling the slack out of the bag.
- Keep the pulling arm straight and the shoulder away from the ear as the slack is pulled from the bag.
- If the hips are twisting or turning, widen the feet a bit.

DUMBBELL ALTERNATING NEUTRAL-GRIP BENCH PRESS

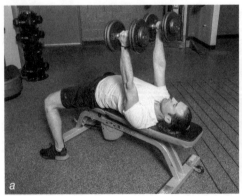 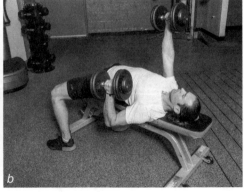

Setup and Performance

- Lie on the back on a flat bench with both feet flat and in a stable position on the ground, holding two dumbbells directly over the shoulders with the arms straight and vertical.
- Grip the dumbbells with the palms facing each other.
- Keep one dumbbell in the top position while lowering the other dumbbell to just above the side of the chest and then push back to the starting position.
- Alternate sides and repeat. One dumbbell will always remain in the top position.

Key Performance Points

- Keep a slight arch in the low back to keep the shoulder blades in the proper depressed and retracted position.
- Drive down through the feet which will provide stability for the push. You may put mats or sturdy plates underneath the feet so they are flat.
- Do not clank the dumbbells together at the top; it is unnecessary unless you enjoy getting paint chips in the eyes.

SPIDERMAN PUSH-UP (ALTERNATING)

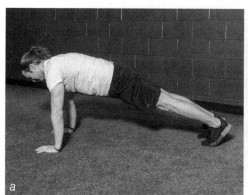 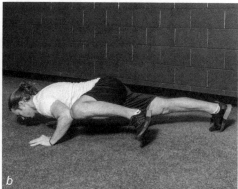

Setup and Performance

- Get into the standard push-up position with the hands slightly wider than shoulder-width apart and the elbows locked out at the top.
- The feet will be hip-width apart.
- In a controlled fashion, lower to the ground keeping the core tight and the elbows at a 45-degree angle from the sides.
- On the descent, simultaneously bring one knee up toward the elbow.
- On the ascent, simultaneously take the foot back to the ground and repeat on the opposite side.

Key Performance Point

- Bringing the leg out to the side adds a rotational stability and hip mobility component to the exercise.

SINGLE-LEG SKATER SQUAT

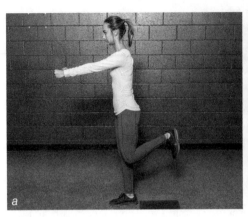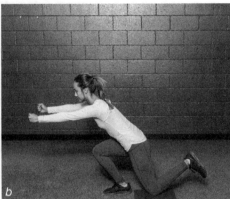

Setup and Performance

- Begin with a pad or elevated box placed directly behind the heels with the feet about hip-width apart.
- Stand on one leg while lifting the opposite leg off the ground. Flex the leg that is in the air by bringing the heel toward the butt.
- Reach the arms out in front of the body making fists. Light dumbbells (5-10 lb [2-5 kg] each) can be held to provide some counterweight if needed.
- Hinge the hips and butt back, descending down toward the pad or box with the knee bent.
- Once the knee lightly touches the pad or box, push through the floor with the stance foot and return to the starting position. Repeat.

Key Performance Points

- The contact made with the pad or box should be a soft touch, a "kiss."
- Create full body tension in this exercise by making tight fists and bracing the core prior to the descent. A lack of tension is a common reason for a lack of success with this movement.
- Only the knee should contact the pad, not the shin.
- Allow a natural forward lean to occur.

KETTLEBELL SIDE-STEP SWING

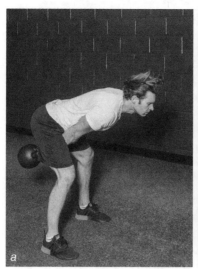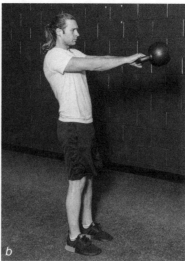

Setup and Performance

- Set a kettlebell 8 to 12 inches in front of the toes with the feet slightly wider than shoulder-width apart.
- Place both hands on the kettlebell handle, tilt the bell back until it forms a straight line with the arms.
- The body position will resemble a starting deadlift position with the hips higher than the knees but lower than the shoulders. Create full-body tension prior to swinging the bell back.
- Hike the bell back keeping the arms between the tops of the legs.
- Push the feet down into the floor and aggressively stand up straight using the hips. The bell will swing forward from the power provided from the hips.
- As the bell swings up, step one foot laterally toward the other foot so that the feet are almost touching when the bell is at chest height and "floating."
- Start to step back out as the bell starts downward into the backswing.
- Complete the backswing and perform continuous swings. Repeat for the designated reps on one side.
- Park the bell safely on the floor when finished with a set of repetitions.

Key Performance Points

- Swings are hip-powered, not arm-powered. This is a key concept to teach.
- Sniff air in on the downswing and hiss air out when the hips extend.
- Keep the spine stable and the arms straight during the swing.
- The body should look like a perfect plank at the top position.

MEDICINE BALL CROSS-BEHIND ROTATIONAL SIDE-SCOOP THROW

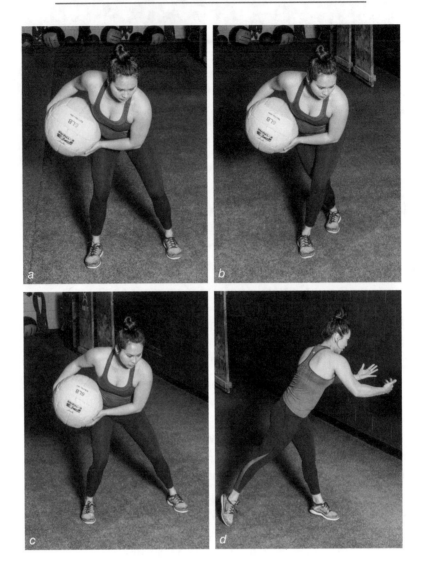

Setup and Performance

- Holding a medicine ball in the hands, turn sideways to the wall and about 10 feet away from it.
- Set the feet a bit wider than shoulder-width apart and push back the hips holding the ball with both hands across the body.
- Perform a cross-behind step (stepping toward wall) with the foot furthest from the wall. Step back out toward the wall with the other foot.
- Simultaneously, sit back and slightly down while turning the shoulders perpendicular to the hips.
- Strongly drive the floor away while rotating open and throw the ball into the wall explosively, turning the hips at the wall on the follow-through.
- Catch the ball, reset, and repeat.

Key Performance Points

- Throw the ball hard; try to break the ball.
- Sit into the hips to properly load them for the throw. The hips are the motor.
- Scoop the ball with both hands as it is thrown at the wall.

DUMBBELL INCLINE SINGLE-ARM BENCH PRESS

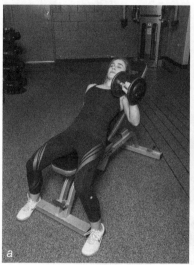 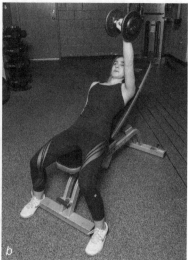

Setup and Performance

- Lie on the back on a incline bench set to about 35-degrees of incline with both feet flat and in a stable position on the ground, holding one dumbbell directly over the shoulder with the arm straight and vertical.
- Use an overhand grip with the palm facing toward the feet.
- Lower the dumbbell to just above the side of the chest and then push back to the starting position.

Key Performance Points

- Keep the shoulder blades down and back throughout the movement.
- Keep a slight arch in the lower back.

SLIDER ECCENTRIC-ONLY SUPINE HIP EXTENSION LEG CURL

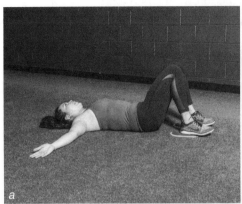
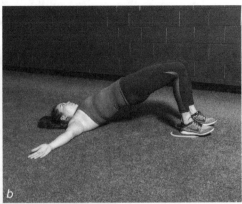
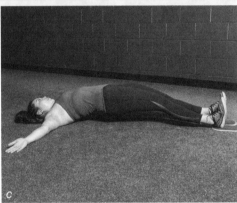

Setup and Performance

- Lie on the floor facing up with the legs straight and the heels placed together on top of a pair of sliders on a sliding surface. Arms are at the sides with the palms up.
- Without lifting the hips, slide the heels toward the butt.
- Set the core and bridge the hips up with the knees bent.
- Slowly extend the knees until the legs are straight. The hips will remain extended and the torso will stay in a straight line from the shoulders, hips, and knees.
- Once the legs are fully straightened, lower the hips to the floor and repeat.

Key Performance Points

- Bracing the core and maintaining the distance between the ribs and hips is critical on this movement to prevent excessive lumbar hyperextension.
- Really fight during the last few inches to get the legs straight before putting the hips on the floor.
- Keep the feet dorsiflexed (feet pulled toward shins) throughout the movement.

CHAPTER 8

Semiprivate and Group Training Programs

Group fitness training has not become popular just recently; these classes have been popular for as long as we can remember. Step, spin, and aerobics classes originated with some of the very first commercial gym models. The social atmosphere is one of the key reasons for the popularity of group training models. As humans, we tend to have a fundamental need to work together and to be a part of something bigger than ourselves (the group or the tribe). Our colleague, Joel Sanders of EXOS, observes that training in a group with like-minded people fosters a "we're in this together" feeling, which is contagious. Developing a sense of comradery is huge, and is another positive aspect of group training that leads to intrinsic (or internal) motivation, which is far more powerful than extrinsic (or external) motivation. In this chapter, we are going to describe how we design general group fitness programs at our gym. If we are trying to optimize a specific client's results, individualized programs are the best option, but group programs are the next best option since price point can frequently be a barrier to entry. Other times, people simply prefer to work in large groups. It is important to have the skills to design effective group programs when those skills are required.

Common Group Fitness Models

As much as any chapter in this book, we need to be very clear with terminology before moving further into the details of programming group fitness training. Let's look at some common group fitness delivery models and establish what they entail:

SEMIPRIVATE (I.E., SMALL GROUP TRAINING)

- Individual programs for each person
- Two to four people in a group with one coach
- Individual programs delivered in a group environment

This is where the terminology can get confusing. Rather than referring to it as *small group training*, we prefer to call this model *semiprivate coaching* to distinguish it from group training and programming in particular. Of course, clients will be working in a small group, but the primary aspect that distinguishes it from large group training is that programming is completely individualized based on each client's goal. You could coach clients from various demographics during the same semiprivate time slot. For example, you may coach a college football player, a grandmother, and a powerlifter, all with different programs and different goals in the same semiprivate training.

...ering individual programs in a group environment requires the coach to work ...p to four individuals during the same class session. The coach does not train ...nts at the same time, but individually coaches each of the clients on his or her ...ogram within the given time period. The secret to success with this model is ...at the coach's attention must be evenly and effectively sprinkled throughout the time block so that everyone has an outstanding coaching experience. What allows us to effectively deliver individual programs in this format is that training sessions all contain the same training components, just different exercises and parameters within those components. So, if we are in the resistance training component, client 1 may be doing a front squat, while client 2 is doing chin-ups, and client 3 is doing push-ups, all within the same approximate time frame.

Some of you may wonder how in the world this can work. You probably have a lot of questions. How do you count their reps? How do you time their rest periods? How do you track their sets? The answer is that you don't. The client tracks what they are capable of tracking. Does a coach need to count the reps for you? We would say no; that's not actually coaching. A coach should be guiding and teaching. Semiprivate training allows for more coaching! The key is that you have to stay proactive and "ABC" (always be coaching), as another colleague, Frank Nash states.

At our facility we don't group our semiprivate clients by abilities, age, training experience, or goals. They group themselves according to the time that want to come in to train. Programming for semiprivate training is done in the same manner as traditional one-on-one or private training. There is no difference in the programming, only in the coaching delivery. The other beauty of this delivery system is that clients still develop the "we're in this together" comradery even though they are working on individual programs.

TEAM TRAINING (LARGE GROUP)

- One program for the group (same for everyone)
- Five or more people in the group with one coach
- The upper limit of coach-to-client ratio determined primarily by logistics, which includes coaching quality

When you reach a certain number of participants in a group, you will no longer be able to deliver individual programs effectively. Experiences with our clientele have shown that this occurs when we exceed the 1:4 coach-to-client ratio. At this point we need to offer only one program to manage the group effectively. The program can be scaled to fit individual clients to a certain degree, but this is when planning and having a solid understanding of exercise progressions and regressions becomes paramount. You also have to be flexible and adept at changing exercises on the fly—there are some inherent trade-offs involved when compared to individualized programming. We feel that group coaching and programming is often more difficult due to all the additional logistics that must be considered. Be prepared, we are going to use the word logistics a lot!

Group Training Logistics

A quick Google search defines *logistics* as "the detailed coordination of a complex operation involving many people, facilities, or supplies." It has become somewhat of an eye-roller to say this word at our gym, but group programming is primarily ruled by logistics. You never want your programming to become logistically undesirable.

This is something to keep in mind when determining if the program you want to implement can be done effectively within the constraints that you have.

The logistics listed here are so variable and different within all gyms that it makes it extremely difficult to give out a lot of absolutes. We will give some examples of what we do as far as some of these logistics are concerned. Here are some logistics to consider when planning for group training:

GROUP GOAL: WHAT IS THE OVERARCHING GOAL?

Most of our clients have the goals of general fat loss and general fitness, so our group model is designed with those in mind, but the group class could certainly be themed differently if there were different group goals. You could create a class theme specifically for powerlifting if that is the group goal, but trying to train someone for powerlifting in a class themed for fat loss wouldn't work too well. Be clear on the stated thematic goal of the class and understand the limitations. Specific goals require specific programming and those goals must be shared in order to effectively program for large groups.

TOTAL TIME AVAILABLE: HOW LONG IS THE SESSION?

Our classes are designed to be completed in approximately 45 minutes, and are capped at 50 minutes. This gives transition time after class, and provides a bit of a buffer.

CLASS SESSION STRUCTURE: HOW IS THE CLASS SESSION ORGANIZED?

To maximize quality training time, here is how we typically organize our time blocks in our group class:

- *Intro/demos*: 5 minutes
- *RAMP*: 10 minutes
- *Metabolic intervals or metabolic resistance and strength training*: 20 to 25 minutes
- *Formal closure*: 2-3 minutes

TOTAL NUMBERS: HOW MANY PEOPLE ARE YOU EXPECTING TO ATTEND, AND WHAT'S THE CAP?

In our space, we plan for 20 people. Typically, we have 8 to 15 people in any given group class, but we plan a for a larger number to be on the safe side.

ROOM SIZE AND SPACE: HOW MUCH SPACE DO YOU HAVE?

Our space for group sessions is about 1600 square feet (148 m²) and fairly open so can we plan accordingly.

EQUIPMENT AVAILABLE: DO YOU HAVE THE TOOLS AVAILABLE FOR THE PLANNED CLASS?

This one is huge. You can't plan for a group of 20 people to do kettlebell swings at the same time if there are only five kettlebells available. You also can't perform alternating bench press and chin-up sets if there is only one power rack and one barbell. The class must be set up differently or other programming choices, such as station work, must be used to maximize the available space and equipment.

TECHNICAL COACHING REQUIRED: HOW MANY HIGHLY COACHING-INTENSIVE EXERCISES DO YOU HAVE GOING ON AT ONE TIME?

In any particular series or circuit, we typically only include one or two highly coaching-intensive exercises at a time due to the inherent challenges of coach ratios in group classes. This sets everyone up for the best opportunity for success. It should be obvious, but it is also critical to only program exercises that you know you can coach competently.

Some other questions that must addressed when planning for group training:

- How will you handle new clients entering the program?
- How will you prescribe and track training loads?
- How many progressions or regressions will be given for an exercise in the session?
- What will you do if a client cannot perform the regression given (or they have common orthopedic concerns)? Do you have a default?

Key Variables and Periodization of Group Fitness Training

The principles of group fat-loss training are the same as the principles that we use for individual fat-loss training that was shared in chapter 4 because it is still based on the principle of our fat-loss training hierarchy. However, by its very nature, planning for group classes has to be more generic or on a global level rather than for the needs of only one. This is one of the inherent compromises with group training. Thus, let's take a look at how we manipulate some of our key programming variables in a group training scenario. Some of the small-picture details change due to previously mentioned logistics and must be considered.

Recall that the fastest way to achieve fat-loss results for the typical time-crunched person in terms of training is:

- two to three resistance training sessions per week, and
- one to two metabolic interval sessions per week.

With this in mind we can design our monthly and weekly group model. At our facility, we offer two different types of classes for our team training members each month. We offer a resistance and strength training class ("Strong" class) and a metabolic interval training class ("Shred" class). Table 8.1 shows a sample of how the class schedule offerings are set up, with details about the Strong and Shred class types to follow.

"Strong" Group Fitness Class

We call our group resistance training classes "Strong," which is the group version of our individually designed resistance training programs for fat loss. For the thematic goal of fat loss, the A and B session full-body training split once again works beautifully here because we serve the needs of the majority while keeping typical time constraints in mind. We also adhere to our traditional hypertrophy rep ranges, working in the 6 to 15 rep range and changing this from month to month. We don't typically use traditionally prescribed sets and reps in this class like we do in our semiprivate programming. Instead, we often use a modified form of density training based on time. Escalating Density Training (EDT) was first introduced to us by Charles Staley and we use a derivative of it in our Strong classes.

EDT is based on the concept that you perform a certain amount of work in a fixed time period. You progress by trying to increase the amount of work done within that same time period, or performing the same work in a shorter time period to increase density. There are a number of ways to implement EDT, but we usually perform a fixed

Table 8.1 Monthly Layout for a Group Fitness Class Session Model

Sunday	Monday	Tuesday	Wednesday	Thursday	Friday	Saturday
1	**2** Holiday	**3** 5 a.m. Shred 4 9 a.m. Shred 4 4:30 p.m. Strong A/B	**4** 5 a.m. Strong A/B 9 a.m. Shred 1 4:30 p.m. Shred 1	**5** 5 a.m. Shred 4 9 a.m. Strong A/B 11 a.m. Shred 4 6 p.m. Shred 4	**6** 5 a.m. Strong A/B 9 a.m. Shred 4	**7** 8 a.m. Shred 2 11 a.m. Shred 4
8	**9** 5 a.m. Strong A/B 9 a.m. Strong A/B 4:30 p.m. Shred 1 6 p.m. Shred 1	**10** 5 a.m. Shred 1 9 a.m. Shred 1 4:30 p.m. Strong A/B	**11** 5 a.m. Strong A/B 9 a.m. Shred 2 4:30 p.m. Shred 2	**12** 5 a.m. Shred 1 9 a.m. Strong A/B 11 a.m. Shred 1 6 p.m. Shred 1	**13** 5 a.m. Strong A/B 9 a.m. Shred 1	**14** 8 a.m. Shred 2 11 a.m. Shred 1
15	**16** 5 a.m. Strong A/B 9 a.m. Strong A/B 4:30 p.m. Shred 2 6 p.m. Shred 2	**17** 5 a.m. Shred 2 9 a.m. Shred 2 4:30 p.m. Strong A/B	**18** 5 a.m. Strong A/B 9 a.m. Shred 3 4:30 p.m. Shred 3	**19** 5 a.m. Shred 2 9 a.m. Strong A/B 11 a.m. Shred 2 6 p.m. Shred 2	**20** 5 a.m. Strong A/B 9 a.m. Shred 2	**21** 8 a.m. Shred 2 11 a.m. Shred 2
22	**23** 5 a.m. Strong A/B 9 a.m. Strong A/B 4:30 p.m. Shred 3 6 p.m. Shred 3	**24** 5 a.m. Shred 3 9 a.m. Shred 3 4:30 p.m. Strong A/B	**25** 5 a.m. Strong A/B 9 a.m. Shred 4 4:30 p.m. Shred 4	**26** 5 a.m. Shred 3 9 a.m. Strong A/B 11 a.m. Shred 3 6 p.m. Shred 3	**27** 5 a.m. Strong A/B 9 a.m. Shred 3	**28** 8 a.m. Shred 2 11 a.m. Shred 3
29	**30** 5 a.m. Strong A/B 9 a.m. Strong A/B 4:30 p.m. Shred 4 6 p.m. Shred 4					

rep count in a circuit of two to four different exercises and do as many quality sets as possible within this time period. See the programs that follow for examples of how this is prescribed. The rest periods are self-selected as needed to keep the quality high. The density approach allows for several different ability levels to attend the same class because loads and work volumes are based on time, and the built-in, autoregulatory nature makes it user- and time-friendly for group strength classes.

The inherent nature of a rank beginner joining a group class, and the various training ages and ability levels in a group class requires a less complex periodization model for the long term. This also makes designing long-term periodization plans logistically undesirable. We compromise by using an alternating linear periodization of reps for our Strong classes over the long term (see table 8.2).

The primary variable that we change in our Strong class each month (it is calendar-based for convenience sake) is repetitions, but you will see in the following programming sections how we manipulate other key variables as well.

Table 8.2 "Strong" Group Fitness Macrocycle: Alternating Linear Periodization of Reps

Month/phase 1: 15 reps	Month/phase 5: 12 reps	Month/phase 9: 10 reps
Month/phase 2: 10 reps	Month/phase 6: 8 reps	Month/phase 10: 6 reps
Month/phase 3: 12 reps	Month/phase 7: 10 reps	Month/phase 11: 12 reps
Month/phase 4: 8 reps	Month/phase 8: 6 reps	Month/phase 12: 8 reps

"Shred" Group Fitness Class

We call our group metabolic interval training classes "Shred," and within a given month, we offer four different formats of this class (we will show some examples in the programming section for this chapter). Our Shred group fitness class is a form of metabolic interval training that is number two in our fat-loss training hierarchy (see chapter 4). We utilize several different delivery protocols in these classes, but these are the general parameters used to create them:

- Total number of highly coaching-intensive exercises per series or circuit will be one to two.
- Total number of exercises in a particular series or circuit will be 1 to 10.
- Total number of different exercises in a single interval session will not be greater than 10.
- Total time of the interval portion (work and rest considered) will be between 20 to 25 minutes.
- Work periods will typically be 20 to 60 seconds.

There are various methods that we use to deliver our interval training protocols with the above parameters. We use the following on a regular basis:

- *Fixed Work, Fixed Recovery*: For example, 30 seconds on and 30 seconds off, or 30 seconds on and 45 seconds off. Recovery can be progressive, meaning it can be increased to allow for the increased fatigue that accumulates. This type of training is based on the clock and is the most common method to prescribe and perform interval work.
- *Fixed Work, Variable Recovery*: For example, 30 seconds on and recover to a pre-determined percentage of estimated maximum heart rate (eMHR), if you have access to heartrate monitors.
- *Variable Work, Variable Recovery*: Work to a predetermined percentage of eMHR and rest to a predetermined percentage of eMHR.

Group Training Programming

Group training, by its very nature, will include varying training ages. Therefore, we will not break down our group programs into the beginner to intermediate and advanced programs since all three levels may be present in one class. Instead, these programs will be combined, and we will describe 12 weeks (or 3 months) of our Strong and Shred classes and how we preplan exercise progressions into our sessions for differing ability levels in one class.

Group Training Program: Month 1, Phase 1

Tables 8.3 through 8.8 show an example of what an actual month of group programming for fat loss would look like in practice at our gym (the tempo key is on page 29). It is important to note that this setup is based on our gym logistics, not yours. The key points to take away are the concepts more so than the exercise specifics. For exercise selection, we provide a primary exercise that would work for 80 percent of the group, plus one progression up and one regression down. One of the unique aspects of general fitness group training is that there may be the full spectrum of training ages participating in the same program, which makes it very challenging to create an effective session for everyone. These preplanned progressions and regressions are limited to three options, which makes this easier on the coach. We have found that in a group environment this design takes a lot of guesswork out of the programming and sets everyone up for success.

Table 8.3 Group Training Month 1/Phase 1 Program: Strong Day A

	Order	Regression exercise	Primary exercise	Progression exercise	Sets/reps	Tempo	Rest
Core training (5 min)	1a.	Incline front plank	Front plank	Suspension trainer front plank	?, 10 min	30-45 sec	?
	1b.		Sandbag alternating birddog isometric hold	Sandbag birddog lateral drag	?, 5 reps each side	3 sec	?
Power development (5 min)	2a.	Medicine ball tall-kneeling forward push throw	Medicine ball forward push throw	Medicine ball forward push throw with alternating step	?, 6 reps (or 3 each side for progression exercise)	X	?
	2b.	Floor ladder forward crossover (slower)	Floor ladder forward crossover	Floor ladder forward crossover (faster)	?, 2 lengths	X	?
Resistance training (10 min)	3a.	Assisted squat	Goblet squat	Two-kettlebell front squat	?, 15 reps	—	?
	3b.		Kettlebell or dumbbell three-point neutral-grip row		?, 15 reps each side	Mod	?
Resistance training (10 min)	4a.	Assisted bodyweight single-leg Romanian deadlift	One-kettlebell or dumbbell staggered-stance Romanian deadlift	One-kettlebell or dumbbell slider single-leg Romanian deadlift	?, 15 reps each side	—	?
	4b.	Incline push-up	Push-up	Suspension trainer push-up	?, 15 reps each side	Mod	?
Regeneration	5.	Supine breathing drill			1 set, 6 breaths	—	?

Note: The number of sets and rest periods are undetermined, so these are designated with a "?". The clients perform as many quality sets as possible in the given time block for each component alternating between the "a" exercise and the "b" exercise. The key to the effectiveness of this approach is to select the proper loads. For the sets of 15 reps, the clients choose a load that would be about a 18RM (rep max).

Table 8.4 Group Training Month 1/Phase 1 Program: Strong Day B

	Order	EXERCISE Regression exercise	Primary exercise	Progression exercise	Sets/reps	Tempo	Rest
Core training (5 min)	1a.	Sandbag side plank from knees	Side plank	Suspension trainer side plank	?, 4-6 reps each side	5 sec	?
	1b.	Sandbag dead bug with alternating 90-degree heel touch	Sandbag dead bug with alternate-leg reach	Sandbag full-dead bug with alternating arm turn	?, 5 reps each side	FE	?
Power development (5 min)	2a.	Medicine ball forward push throw	Medicine ball floor slam	Medicine ball rotational floor slam	?, 6 reps (or 3 each side for progression exercise)	X	?
	2b.	Floor ladder forward two in/two out (slower)	Floor ladder forward two in/two out	Floor ladder forward two in/two out (faster)	?, 2 lengths	X	?
Resistance training (10 min)	3a.	Prisoner bodyweight Romanian deadlift	Kettlebell deadlift	Two-kettlebell deadlift	?, 15 reps	—	?
	3b.	Push-up	Kettlebell or dumbbell single-arm floor press	Kettlebell or dumbbell single-arm bench press	? x 15 each side (15 reps total for regression exercise)	Mod	?
Resistance training (10 min)	4a.	Assisted bottoms-up split squat	Goblet split squat	Two-kettlebell or dumbbell split squat	?, 15 reps each side	—	?
	4b.		Suspension trainer inverted neutral-grip row		?, 15 reps	Mod	?
Regeneration	5.	Supine breathing drill			1 set, 6 breaths	—	—

Note: The number of sets and rest periods are undetermined so these are designated with a "?". The clients perform as many quality sets as possible in the given time block for each component alternating between the "a" exercise and the "b" exercise. The key to the effectiveness of this approach is to select the proper loads. For the sets of 15 reps, to the clients choose a load that would be about a 18RM (rep max).

Table 8.5   Group Training Month 1/Phase 1 Program: Shred 1

These are time-based circuits in which each station occurs at the same time for three rounds. Rounds 1 and 2 are 30 seconds on and 30 seconds off with a six-second transition between partner exchanges and stations. Round 3 is 15 seconds on and 15 seconds off with a six-second transition between partner exchanges and stations.

Order	EXERCISE		
	Regression exercise	Primary exercise	Progression exercise
1a.		Fan bikes, treadmill sprints, or stair climber machines	
1b.		Medicine ball forward push throw (from base position)	Medicine ball forward push throw + squat thrust
1c.	Suspension trainer assisted squat	Bodyweight speed squat	Prisoner vertical jump(continuous)
1d.	Medicine ball rotational side throw	Medicine ball rotational side throw with step	Medicine ball alternating rotational side throw
1e.	Two-kettlebell push press	Two-kettlebell piston push press	Two-kettlebell front squat and press
1f.	Sandbag high pull	Kettlebell swing	Kettlebell side-step swing
1g.		Battling rope snap (various patterns)	
1h.	Suspension trainer alternating reverse lunge	Sandbag front reverse lunge up-down	Sandbag alternating rotational reverse lunge
1i.	Medicine ball modified squat thrust	Medicine ball squat thrust	Medicine ball burpee
2 min rest; coaching instruction			

Table 8.6   Group Training Month 1/Phase 1 Program: Shred 2

These are circuits in which the clients work to 85 to 95 percent eMHR, recover to 70 percent eMHR, then go to the next exercise for three nine-minute rounds.

Order	EXERCISE		
	Regression exercise	Primary exercise	Progression exercise
1a.	Suspension trainer alternating reverse lunge	Suspension trainer alternating split-squat jump	Alternating split-squat jump
1b.	Medicine ball side throw	Medicine ball alternating rotational side throw	
1c.	Kettlebell swing	Kettlebell single-arm swing	Kettlebell single-arm snatch
2 min rest; coaching instruction			
2a.	Medicine ball chest throw	Medicine ball front squat + chest throw	
2b.		Bikes *or* Woodway curve sprint *or* Stepmill *or* jump rope	
2c.	Rope alternating wave	Rope squatting alternating wave	
2 min rest; coaching instruction			
3a.	Medicine ball floor slam	Medicine ball rollover floor slam	
3b.		Floor ladder forward crossover	
3c.	Medicine ball modified squat thrust	Medicine ball squat thrust	Medicine ball burpee

Table 8.7 Group Training Month 1/Phase 1 Program: Shred 3

These are circuits in which the clients perform the first exercise to 85 to 90 percent eMHR and recover to 75 to 80 percent eMHR, then perform next exercise to 85 to 90 percent eMHR and recover to 70 percent eMHR, repeating this pattern through all exercises. This is repeated for four six-minute rounds.

| Order | EXERCISE | | |
	Regression exercise	Primary exercise	Progression exercise
1a.	Medicine ball forward push throw	Medicine ball floor slam	Medicine ball rotational floor slam
1b.		Bikes *or* Woodway curve sprint *or* alternating speed step-up *or* jump rope	
2a.	Suspension trainer alternating reverse lunge	Suspension trainer split-squat jump	Split-squat jump
2b.		Bikes *or* Woodway curve sprint *or* alternating speed step-up *or* jump rope	
3a.	Sandbag clean	Sandbag clean + push press	Sandbag alternating lateral-step Romanian deadlift–clean
3b.	Medicine ball modified squat thrust	Medicine ball mountain climber	Mountain climber
4a.		Rope interval (pattern of choice; change pattern every 10 sec)	
4b.		Floor ladder two-in/one-out shuffle	

Table 8.8 Group Training Month 1/Phase 1 Program: Shred 4

These are circuits in which the clients work to 85 to 95 percent eMHR and recover to 70 percent eMHR, repeating this pattern for each block of time. This is repeated for eight three-minute rounds. If numbers allow, each participant does the same exercise at the same time.

| Order | EXERCISE | | |
	Regression exercise	Primary exercise	Progression exercise
1.	Medicine ball floor slam	Medicine ball floor slam + hand walk-out	
2.	Sandbag alternating reverse lunge up-down	Sandbag alternating reverse lunge	
3.		Rip trainer low slap shot	Rip trainer low-medium-high slap shot
4.	Kettlebell hike	Kettlebell swing	Kettlebell hand-to-hand swing
5.	Medicine ball floor slam	Medicine ball floor slam + hand walk-out	
6.	Sandbag alternating reverse lunge up-down	Sandbag alternating rotational reverse lunge	
7.		Rip trainer low slap shot	Rip trainer low-medium-high slap shot
8.	Kettlebell hike	Kettlebell swing	Kettlebell hand-to-hand swing

Group Training Program: Month 2/Phase 2

Phase 2 continues where phase 1 left off. Notice that we move to 10 reps sets for in our rep programming for our Strong day A and day B in the resistance training component. We also change the parameters in how we deliver our metabolic training to keep that aspect fresh and exciting. See tables 8.9 through 8.14 for examples of group training programs for phase 2.

Table 8.9 Group Training Month 2/Phase 2 Program: Strong, Day A

	Order	EXERCISE			Sets/reps	Tempo	Rest
		Regression exercise	Primary exercise	Progression exercise			
Core training (5 min)	1a.	Side plank	Suspension trainer side plank	Side plank + band single-arm row	?, 1 rep each side (with 10 rows each side for progression exercise)	20-30 sec	?
	1b.	Sandbag unsupported leg-lowering (6 each side)	Suspension trainer prone jack-knife	Suspension trainer prone pike	?, 6-8 reps (6 each side for regression exercise)	1-2-1	?
Power development (5 min)	Order	Regression exercise	Primary exercise	Progression exercise	Sets/reps	Tempo	Rest
	2a.	Medicine ball chest throw from base position	Medicine ball side throw	Medicine ball cross-behind side scoop throw	?, 5 reps each side (10 reps for regression exercise)	X	?
	2b.	Floor ladder lateral two-in/two-out (slower)	Floor ladder lateral two-in/two-out	Floor ladder lateral two-in/two-out (faster)	?, 1 length each direction	X	?
Resistance training (10 min)	Order	Regression exercise	Primary exercise	Progression exercise	Sets/reps	Tempo	Rest
	3a.	One-kettlebell or dumbbell slider single-leg Romanian deadlift	One-kettlebell or dumbbell single-leg Romanian deadlift (contra)	Two-kettlebell or dumbbell single-leg deadlift	?, 10 reps each side	—	?
	3b.	Incline push-up	Push-up	Suspension trainer push-up	?, 10 reps	Mod	?
Resistance training (10 min)	4a.	Assisted squat	Goblet squat	Two-kettlebell front squat	?, 10 reps	—	?
	4b.		Kettlebell or dumbbell three-point neutral-grip row	Dumbbell two-point single-leg neutral-grip row	?, 10 reps each side	Mod	?
Regeneration	5.	Suspension trainer squat hang breathing drill			1 set, 6 breaths	—	—

Note: The number of sets and the rest periods are undetermined and designated with a "?". The clients perform as many quality sets as possible in the given time block for each component alternating between the "a" and "b" exercises. The key to the effectiveness of this approach is to select the proper loads. For the sets of 10 reps in the resistance component, the clients choose a load that would be about a 12-13RM (rep max).

Table 8.10 Group Training Month 2/Phase 2 Program: Strong Day B

	Order	EXERCISE Regression exercise	Primary exercise	Progression exercise	Sets/reps	Tempo	Rest
Core training (5 min)	1a.	Front plank	Suspension trainer front plank	Suspension trainer body saw	?, 1 rep (6-8 total for progression exercise)	30-45 sec	?
	1b.	Sandbag alternating birddog isometric hold	Sandbag birddog lateral drag	Sandbag alternating bear with isometric hold	?, 5 reps each side	Slow	?
	Order	EXERCISE Regression exercise	Primary exercise	Progression exercise	Sets/reps	Tempo	Rest
Power development (5 min)	2a.	Medicine ball floor slam	Medicine ball rotational floor slam		?, 3 reps each side (6 total for regression exercise)	X	?
	2b.	Floor ladder forward wide-out (slower)	Floor ladder forward wide-out	Floor ladder forward wide-out (faster)	?, 2 lengths	X	?
	Order	EXERCISE Regression exercise	Primary exercise	Progression exercise	Sets/reps	Tempo	Rest
Resistance training (10 min)	3a.	Assisted bottoms-up split squat	Goblet split squat	Two-kettlebell or dumbbell split squat	?, 10 reps each side	—	?
	3b.		Suspension trainer inverted neutral-grip row	Band-assisted chin-up	?, 10 reps (5-10 total for progression exercise)	Mod	?
Resistance training (10 min)	4a.	Kettlebell deadlift	Two-kettlebell deadlift	High hex bar deadlift	?, 10 reps	—	?
	4b.	Landmine kneeling single-arm press *or* Kettlebell single-arm floor press	Kettlebell kneeling single-arm overhead press	Kettlebell single-arm overhead press	?, 10 reps each side	—	?
Regeneration	5.	Suspension trainer squat hang breathing drill			1 set, 6 breaths	_	?

Note: The number of sets and the rest periods are undetermined and designated with a "?". The clients perform as many quality sets as possible in the given time block for each component alternating between the "a" and "b" exercises. The key to the effectiveness of this approach is to select the proper loads. For the sets of 10 reps in the resistance components, the clients choose a load that would be about a 12RM-13RM (rep max).

Table 8.11 Group Training Month 2/Phase 2 Program: Shred 1

These are circuits in which the clients complete each circuit or complex and recover to 70 percent eMHR, repeating this pattern for each block of time before moving to the next complex or circuit. This is repeated for four total five-to-six-minute rounds.

Order	Exercise
1.	Medicine ball circuit: •Medicine ball floor slam, 10 •Medicine ball forward push throw, 10 •Medicine ball burpee, 10 (modified squat thrust for regression)
2.	Sandbag complex: •Sandbag high pull, 5 •Sandbag bent-over row, 5 •Sandbag push press, 5 •Sandbag lateral-step Romanian deadlift and clean (or high pull), 5 each side
3.	Kettlebell complex: •Kettlebell swing, 15 •Kettlebell deadlift, 10 •Kettlebell goblet squat, 5
4.	Medicine ball circuit: •Medicine ball alternating side throw, 10 each side •Medicine ball mountain climber, 10 •Medicine ball front squat, 10

Table 8.12 Group Training Month 2/Phase 2 Program: Shred 2

These are circuits in which the clients work to 85 to 90 percent eMHR, recover to 70 percent eMHR, then perform the next exercise in the circuit for the designated block of time. This is repeated for two 11 to 12 minute rounds.

Order	Exercise
1a.	Air assault sprint *or* Woodway curve sprint *or* Stepmill
1b.	Medicine ball alternating shot put throw
1c.	Alternating low-lateral step-up (air assault for regression)
1d.	Battling ropes (various patterns)
2 min rest; coaching instruction	
2a.	Medicine ball front squat + floor slam + forward push throw
2b.	Sandbag rotational clean
2c.	Air assault sprint *or* Woodway curve sprint *or* Stepmill
2d.	Kettlebell swing (kettlebell hike for regression; kettlebell single-arm swing for progression)

Table 8.13 Group Training Month 2/Phase 2 Program: Shred 3

These are time-based circuits in which each station occurs at the same time for two to three rounds, where round 1 is 30 seconds on and 30 seconds off, round 2 is 30 seconds on and 40 seconds off, and round 3 is 30 seconds on and 50 seconds off.

Order	Exercise
1a.	Floor ladder forward crossover
1b.	Rip trainer low slap shot
1c.	Suspension trainer rotational single-arm row (suspension trainer single-arm row for regression)
1d.	Sandbag alternating lateral step Romanian deadlift with high pull
1e.	Medicine ball shot put throw
1f.	Suspension trainer jump squat (bodyweight speed squat for regression; prisoner vertical jump for progression)
1g.	Air assault sprint *or* Woodway curve sprint *or* Stepmill
1h.	Slam ball snatch + floor slam
2 min rest; coaching instruction	

Table 8.14 Group Training Month 2/Phase 2 Program: Shred 4

These are circuits in which the clients work to 85 to 95 percent eMHR, recover to 70 percent eMHR, then go to the next exercise in the circuit for the designated block of time. There are three nine-minute rounds.

Order	EXERCISE		
	Regression exercise	Primary exercise	Progression exercise
1a.		Rope interval (pattern of choice; change pattern every 10 sec)	
1b.		Bikes *or* Woodway curve sprint *or* Step mill *or* jump rope	
1c.	Medicine ball rotational side throw	Medicine ball alternating rotational side throw	
2 min rest; coaching instruction			
2a.	Kettlebell hike	Kettlebell swing	Kettlebell side-step swing
2b.	Medicine ball chest throw + floor slam	Medicine ball front squat + floor slam	
2c.	Assisted lateral lunge	Bodyweight alternating lateral lunge	
2 min rest; coaching instruction			
3a.	Alternating reverse lunge	Sandbag alternating rotational reverse lunge	Sandbag alternating rotational forward and reverse lunge
3b.		Medicine ball forward push throw	
3c.		Rope grappler twist	

Group Training Program: Month 3/Phase 3

In phase 3, the metabolic presentation parameters change once again, increasing to 12 rep sets for the resistance training component. Tables 8.15 through 8.20 show examples of group training programs for phase 3.

Table 8.15   Group Training Month 3/Phase 3 Program: Strong Day A

	Order	EXERCISE Regression exercise	Primary exercise	Progression exercise	Sets/reps	Tempo	Rest
Core training (5 min)	1a.	Suspension trainer front plank	Suspension trainer body saw	Suspension trainer kneeling fallout	?, 6-8 reps	Slow	?
	1b.	Sandbag birddog lateral drag	Sandbag alternating bear with isometric hold	Sandbag bear lateral drag	?, 5 reps each side	Slow	?
	Order	EXERCISE Regression exercise	Primary exercise	Progression exercise	Sets/reps	Tempo	Rest
Power development (5 min)	2.	Kettlebell hike	Kettlebell dead swing	Kettlebell swing	5 sets, 8 reps	X	45 sec
	Order	EXERCISE Regression exercise	Primary exercise	Progression exercise	Sets/reps	Tempo	Rest
Resistance training (10 min)	3a.	Goblet squat	Kettlebell single-arm front squat (alternate sides each set)	Kettlebell single-arm tempo front squat (alternate sides each set)	?, 12 reps	3-1-3 for progression exercise	?
	3b.	Kettlebell or dumbbell three-point neutral-grip row	Suspension trainer single-arm row	Suspension trainer rotational single-arm row	?, 12 reps each side	—	?
Resistance training (10 min)	4a.	One-kettlebell or dumbbell slider single-leg Romanian deadlift	One-kettlebell or dumbbell single-leg Romanian deadlift (contra)	Two-kettlebell or dumbbell single-leg deadlift	?, 12 reps each side	—	?
	4b.	Push-up	Single-leg push-up	T-push-up	?, 6 reps each side (12 total for regression exercise)	—	?
Regeneration	5.	Wall 90-90 breathing drill			1 set, 6 breaths	—	—

Note: The number of sets and the rest periods are undetermined and designated with a "?". The clients will perform as many quality sets as possible in the given time block for each component alternating between the "a" and "b" exercises. The key to the effectiveness of this approach is to select the proper loads. For the sets of 12 reps in the resistance components, the clients choose a load that would be about a 15RM (rep max).

Table 8.16 Group Training Month 3/Phase 3 Program: Strong Day B

	Order	EXERCISE Regression exercise	Primary exercise	Progression exercise	Sets/reps	Tempo	Rest
Core training (5 min)	1a.	Side plank + band single-arm row	Kettlebell or dumbbell single-arm farmer's walk (switch sides after 20 yd)	Kettlebell single-arm bottoms-up rack walk (switch sides after 20 yd)	?, 20 yd each side (10 each side for regression exercise)	—	?
	1b.	Suspension trainer prone jackknife	Suspension trainer prone pike	Hanging knee raise	?, 6-8 reps (3-5 for progression exercise)	Slow	?
Power development (5 min)		EXERCISE Regression exercise	Primary exercise	Progression exercise	Sets/reps	Tempo	Rest
	2a.	Medicine ball side throw	Medicine ball shot put throw	Medicine ball cross-behind shot put throw	?, 5 reps each side	X	?
	2b.	Drop to base	Box jump	Prisoner vertical jump	?, 5 reps	X	?
Resistance training (10 min)		EXERCISE Regression exercise	Primary exercise	Progression exercise	Sets/reps	Tempo	Rest
	3a.	Kettlebell deadlift	Kettlebell single-arm deadlift (alternate sides each set)	Kettlebell tempo deadlift (alternate sides each set)	?, 12 reps	— (3-1-3 for progression exercise)	?
	3b.	Kettlebell single-arm floor press	Kettlebell single-arm overhead press	Kettlebell alternating overhead press	?, 12 reps each side	—	?
Resistance training (10 min)	4a.	Goblet split squat	Goblet reverse lunge	Goblet cross-behind lunge	?, 12 reps each side	—	?
	4b.	Suspension trainer inverted neutral-grip row	Band-assisted chin-up	Chin-up	?, 10 reps (12 for regression exercise)	Mod	?
Regeneration	5.	Wall 90-90 breathing drill			1 set, 6 breaths	—	—

Note: The number of sets and the rest periods are undetermined and designated with a "?". The clients perform as many quality sets as possible in the given time block for each component alternating between the "a" and "b" exercises. The key to the effectiveness of this approach is to select the proper loads. For the sets of 12 reps in the resistance components, the clients choose a load that would be about a 15RM (rep max).

Table 8.17   Group Training Month 3/Phase 3 Program: Shred 1

These are circuits in which the clients work to 85 to 95 percent eMHR, recover to 70 percent eMHR, then go to the next exercise in the circuit for the designated block of time. There are three rounds in which the first round is 10 minutes, the second round is 8 minutes, and the third round is 6 minutes.

Order	Exercise
1a.	Air Assault sprint *or* Woodway curve sprint *or* jump rope
1b.	Medicine ball floor slam
1c.	Sandbag alternating front and reverse lunge up-down
1d.	Floor ladder lateral two-in/two-out
2 min rest; coaching instruction	
2a.	Sandbag complex: Sandbag staggered-stance bent-over row, 5 each side Sandbag clean + push press, 10
2b.	Medicine ball cross-behind side throw (medicine ball side throw for regression)
2c.	Rope alternating wave (rope squatting alternating wave for progression)
2 min rest; coaching instruction	
3a.	Kettlebell swing (kettlebell dead swing for regression; kettlebell snatch for progression)
3b.	Medicine ball front squat + chest throw + squat thrust

Table 8.18   Group Training Month 3/Phase 3 Program: Shred 2

For these time-based circuits, the first group of exercises is performed 30 seconds on and 30 seconds off for two rounds; the second group is performed 30 seconds on and 40 seconds off for two rounds; and the third group is performed 30 seconds on and 50 seconds off for two rounds.

Order	EXERCISE		
	Regression exercise	Primary exercise	Progression exercise
1a.		Bikes *or* Woodway curve sprint *or* Stepmill *or* jump rope	
1b.		Medicine ball shot put throw	Medicine ball alternating shot put throw
1c.		Sandbag alternating front and reverse lunge up-down	Sandbag front up-down + overhead press
2 min rest; coaching instruction			
2a.	Sandbag clean	Sandbag clean + press	Sandbag clean + rotational press
2b.	Medicine ball modified squat thrust	Medicine ball squat thrust	Medicine ball burpee
2c.		Medicine ball forward push throw	
2 min rest; coaching instruction			
3a.	Rope (pattern of choice)	Rope alternating wave	Rope squatting alternating wave
3b.	Kettlebell hike	Kettlebell swing	Kettlebell single-arm swing
3c.		Floor ladder (variation of choice)	

Table 8.19   Group Training Month 3/Phase 3 Program: Shred 3

These are circuits in which the clients work to 85 to 95 percent eMHR, recover to 70 percent eMHR, then go to the next exercise in the circuit for the designated block of time. There are two 10 to 12-minute rounds.

| Order | EXERCISE | | |
	Regression exercise	Primary exercise	Progression exercise
1a.	Medicine ball modified squat thrust	Medicine ball squat thrust	Medicine ball burpee
1b.	Sandbag clean + bent-over row	Sandbag clean + push press	Sandbag rotational clean + push press
1c.	Floor ladder lateral in-in/out-out (slower)	Floor ladder lateral in-in/out-out	Floor ladder lateral in-in/out-out (faster)
1d.		Battling rope in-out wave	
1e.		Fan bike *or* VersaClimber	
2 min rest; coaching instruction			
2a.	Kettlebell swing	Kettlebell single-arm swing	Kettlebell snatch
2b.		Medicine ball side throw	
2c.	Floor ladder (pattern of choice)	Floor ladder forward 1-2-3	
2d.		Medicine ball floor slam + side throw (10 each side)	
2e.	Assisted or bodyweight alternating reverse lunge	Sandbag alternating front and reverse lunge up-down	Sandbag alternating rotational reverse lunge

Table 8.20   Group Training Month 3/Phase 3 Program: Shred 4

These are time-based circuits in which each station occurs at the same time for three rounds. Round 1 is 40 seconds on and 40 seconds off, round 2 is 30 seconds on and 30 seconds off, and round 3 is 20 seconds on and 20 seconds off. There is a six second transition between partner exchanges and stations for all rounds.

| Order | EXERCISE | | |
	Regression exercise	Primary exercise	Progression exercise
1a.	Medicine ball modified squat thrust	Medicine ball squat thrust	Medicine ball burpee
1b.	Medicine ball chest throw from base position	Medicine ball rotational side throw	Medicine ball alternating rotational side throw
1c.	Sandbag alternating lateral-step Romanian deadlift	Sandbag alternating lateral-step Romanian deadlift with clean	Sandbag alternating lateral-step Romanian deadlift with overhead chop
1d.	Rope alternating wave	Rope alternating wave with alternating side step	
1e.		Medicine ball floor slam	Medicine ball alternating side-step slam
1f.	Kettlebell swing	Kettlebell single-arm swing	Kettlebell single-arm snatch
1g.	Assisted or bodyweight alternating reverse lunge	Sandbag alternating front and reverse lunge up-down	Sandbag alternating rotational reverse lunge
1h.		Air assault sprint *or* Woodway curve sprint *or* Stepmill	
2 min rest; coaching instruction			

SELECT GROUP FITNESS PROGRAM EXERCISES

MEDICINE BALL FORWARD PUSH THROW WITH ALTERNATING STEP

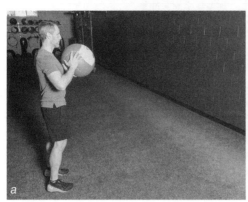 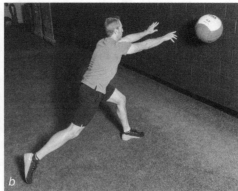

Setup and Performance

- Start by facing about 10 feet back from a solid brick wall, holding a medicine ball at chest height with the feet about hip-width apart.
- Rise up on the toes and keep the body in a straight line while falling forward toward the wall.
- Step out and forward with one foot to catch oneself while simultaneously pushing the ball into the wall as hard and fast as possible. Reset and repeat, stepping forward with the opposite foot on the next repetition.

Key Performance Point

- Sound is a great tool for feedback. Throw the ball hard; try to "break" the ball.

FLOOR LADDER FORWARD CROSSOVER

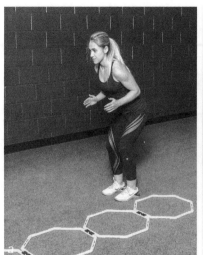 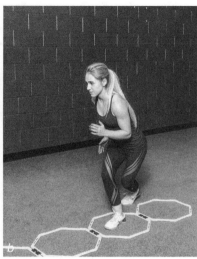

Setup and Performance

- Stand on the right-hand side of the ladder facing forward, and step into the first ladder rung with the right foot.
- Step back out and slightly forward to the other side of the ladder with the left foot and then the right foot again. Both feet will be on the opposite side of the ladder at this point.
- Next, start with the left foot and repeat the same pattern moving up the length of the ladder with the appropriate speed.

Key Performance Point

- Perform the pattern slowly at first and then work to move faster.

SANDBAG FULL-DEAD BUG WITH ALTERNATING ARM TURN

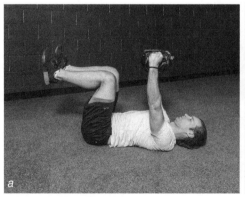 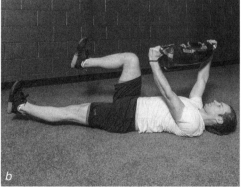

Setup and Performance

- Lie on the back and bring the legs up into a 90-degree hip and knee flexed position.
- Hold the sandbag by the outside handles over the chest with the wrists straight and the arms fully extended.
- Pull the handles of the bag apart and bring the ribs down to slightly press the low back into the floor.
- Maintaining the pelvic position, extend one leg so that it hovers slightly off the ground.
- Simultaneously, as the leg extends, rotate the bag so that the opposing arm's hand is the top hand relative to the head.
- Fully exhale at this position. Simultaneously bring the arms and legs back to the starting position and repeat on the other side.

Key Performance Points

- Be sure to pull the handles of the sandbag apart while extending the leg. This will help create and maintain top-down body tension and pelvic stability. Prevent the bag from sagging.
- Reset the tension between each rep.

MEDICINE BALL ROTATIONAL FLOOR SLAM

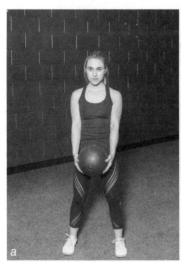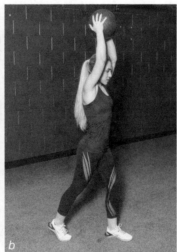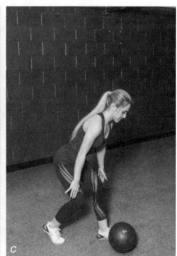

Setup and Performance

- Stand with the feet about shoulder-width apart, holding a medicine ball (ideally a non-bouncing medicine ball) at hip height.
- Bring the ball overhead and rotate at the hips and shoulders, slamming the ball down on the ground on one side, slightly in front of the body.
- Pick up the ball and repeat on the other side for the designated sets and reps.

Key Performance Points

- Brace the core strongly to prevent the ribs and hips from being separated.
- Load the hips to prepare to throw the medicine ball.
- Allow the back heel to come up as the ball is thrown to allow the hips to fully release.

KETTLEBELL SINGLE-ARM FLOOR PRESS

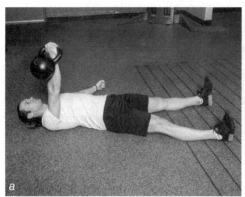 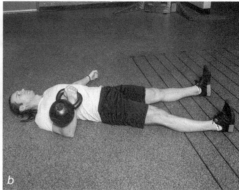

Setup and Performance

- Lie on the back on the floor with both legs straight and one kettlebell directly over the shoulder with the arm straight and vertical.
- Lower the kettlebell so that the upper arm touches the floor just above the side of the chest and then push back to the starting position. Repeat and switch sides.

Key Performance Points

- At the bottom of the movement the upper arm will be about 45 degrees from the torso.
- Keep the shoulder blades down and back throughout the movement.
- Hold the kettlebell deep in the palm so that the wrist stays straight and neutral.

PRISONER VERTICAL JUMP (CONTINUOUS)

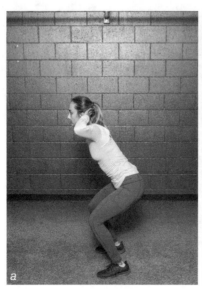 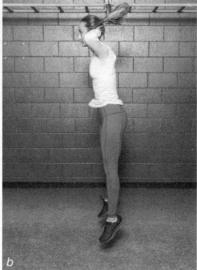

Setup and Performance

- Begin in a stance that will allow the highest jump. Typically, this will be with the feet about hip-width apart or slightly wider.

- Interlace the fingers and place the hands behind the head in the "prisoner" position. Lower the hips down to quarter-squat depth and jump as high as possible. Land under control, absorbing the force and immediately go into the next jump and repeat.

Key Performance Points

- This is commonly called a squat jump but we call it a vertical jump because you don't actually perform a full squat when you attempt to jump for maximal height.
- Perform these repetitions continuously rather than one at a time, with a reset between each rep.

SANDBAG ALTERNATING ROTATIONAL REVERSE LUNGE

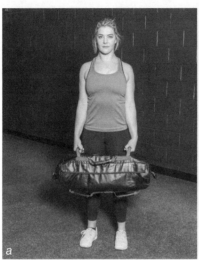 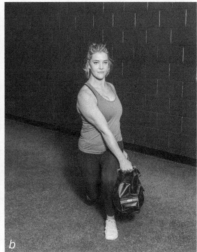

Setup and Performance

- Stand with feet about hip-width apart holding a sandbag in front of the body with the arms straight and the hands holding the neutral-grip handles.
- Step back with one foot and drop into a reverse lunge and bring the bag over the forward leg.
- Push through both feet back to the top and seamlessly perform a repetition to the other side. Keep alternating sides as needed.

Key Performance Points

- The rotation in this movement is from the bag rotating around the body; it comes from the thoracic spine and shoulders not the lumbar spine.
- Keep the belly button pointed forward.
- Keep the eyes forward.

MEDICINE BALL BURPEE

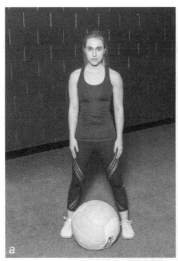 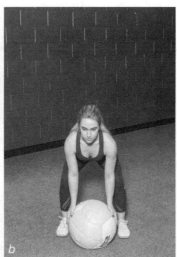 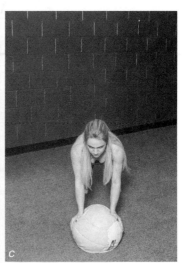

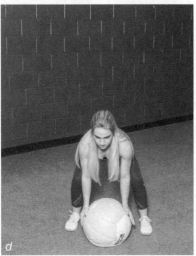 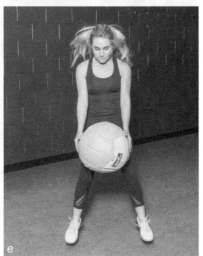

Setup and Performance

- Stand with the feet slightly wider than shoulder-width apart and place a medicine ball between the feet.
- Bend down in a squatting motion and place the hands on top of the ball. Jump the feet back together and then jump the feet back up to where they started.
- Immediately upon coming back up, hold onto the medicine ball and perform a vertical jump.
- Land softly and repeat the movements.

Key Performance Points

- Keep the hands stacked under the shoulders.
- The purpose of the medicine ball is to provide some extra space so that the spine can be kept in good alignment; a box can also be used.
- The jump can be omitted if needed (which we call a squat thrust), and one can step the legs out and back one at a time if needed (which we call a modified squat thrust).

KETTLEBELL SINGLE-ARM SNATCH

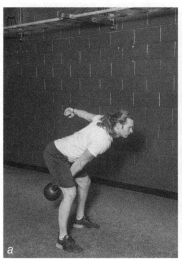 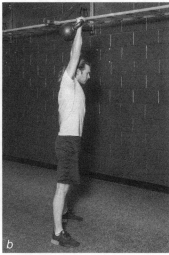

Setup and Performance

- Set the kettlebell 8 to 12 inches (20-30 cm) in front of the toes with the feet slightly wider than shoulder-width apart.
- Place one hand on the kettlebell handle; tilt the bell back so it forms a straight line with the arms.
- The body position will resemble a starting deadlift position with the hips higher than the knees but lower than the shoulders. Create full-body tension prior to swinging the bell back.
- Hike the bell back keeping the arm above the knees.
- Push the feet down into the floor and aggressively stand up straight using the hips. The bell will swing forward from the power provided from the hips.
- The snatch differs from the one-arm swing in that it is a short tight arc on the upswing as opposed to the long arc of the swing. Once the bell passes the hips on the upswing of the snatch, the elbow bends and the arc becomes more vertical.
- Punch through the kettlebell at the top so that the bell lands softly on the back of the forearm.
- From the top position, reverse the actions remembering to keep the kettlebell fairly close to the body.
- Guide the kettlebell back so that the force is absorbed with the hips.
- Perform continuous snatches and repeat for the designated time or repetitions.

Key Performance Points

- The most common mistake in performing the kettlebell snatch is keeping the arm straight the during the entire motion. This also contributes to the dreaded banging and bruising of the forearm at the catch position. You will not be able to "tame the arc" (to quote Pavel Tsatsouline) properly unless you bend the arm at the correct time, which is in the second part of the upswing and the first part of the downswing.
- Be sure the client is prepared to perform snatches and that you are prepared to coach them. Never program exercises that you are unprepared to coach. The client must have a solid foundation of single-arm swings and be cleared to go overhead.
- Snatches are hip-powered, not arm-powered. This is a key concept to teach and understand.
- Sniff in the air on the downswing and hiss out the air when the hips extend.
- Keep the shoulders relatively square in the backswing position.

ROPE SQUATTING ALTERNATING WAVE

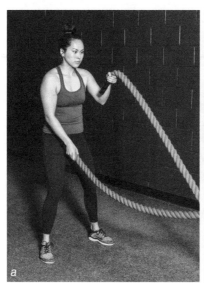
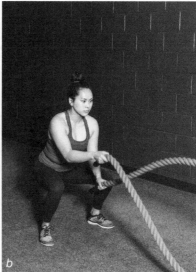

Setup and Performance

- Stand in an athletic stance holding the ends of a battling rope that is anchored to the ground.
- Find the sweet-spot distance from the anchor that allows you to use as much velocity as possible. Don't be too far forward or too far back.
- Start making whippy alternating waves in the rope while simultaneously performing a squatting motion.

Key Performance Points

- Keep the neck in a neutral position rather than in a flexed position.
- Don't pull back on the ropes; instead, whip them up and down as if holding large drumsticks and beating on a large drum.

SANDBAG ALTERNATING LATERAL-STEP ROMANIAN DEADLIFT–CLEAN

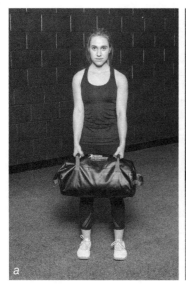
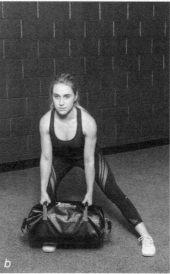
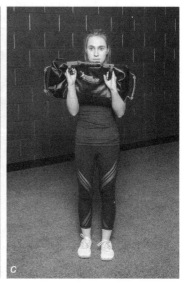

Setup and Performance

- Stand with the feet about hip-width apart holding a sandbag in front of the body with the arms straight and the hands holding the neutral-grip handles.
- Step out to the side with one foot and hip hinge into the stepping leg. The trailing leg will be straight and the sandbag will be in front of the stepping leg.
- Load the hip and immediately push back to the starting-foot position performing a sandbag clean, catching the bag in the crooks of the elbows.
- Step out to the opposite side while at the same time unwinding the bag, and seamlessly perform a repetition to the other side. Keep alternating sides as required.

Key Performance Points

- Keep the bag close to the body at all times on the clean portion of the movement.
- The clean is hip-powered and not arm-powered.

MEDICINE BALL MOUNTAIN CLIMBER

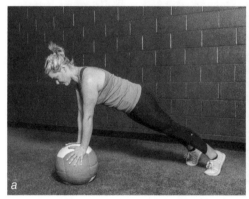 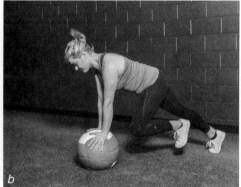

Setup and Performance

- Place a large medicine ball on the ground and get into a tall plank position with the hand on the ball.
- Bring one leg up into a hip-and-knee-flexed position.
- Keeping the spine and hip stable, alternate driving the legs up and back in a piston-like motion for the designated time or repetitions.

Key Performance Points

- The purpose of the medicine ball is to provide some extra space so that the spine can be kept in good alignment, a box can also be used.
- Keep the shoulders and hips in line with each other.
- Keep the hands stacked under the shoulders.

MEDICINE BALL FLOOR SLAM AND HAND WALK-OUT

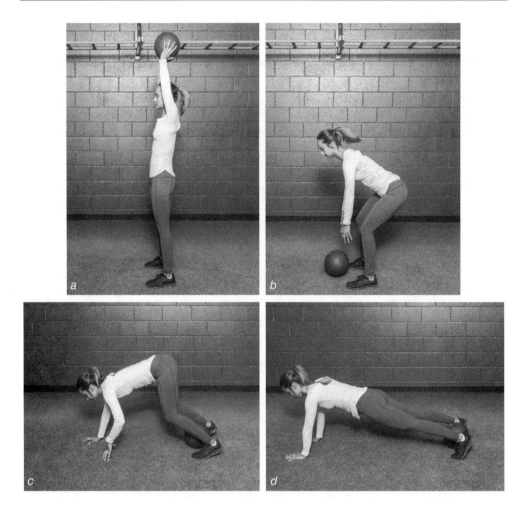

Setup and Performance

- Stand with the feet about shoulder-width apart, holding a medicine ball (ideally a non-bouncing medicine ball) at hip height.
- Bring the ball overhead and slam the ball down on the ground just in front of the feet.
- Stand and then hip hinge to bend over and place the hands on the floor.
- Walk the hands out to a top of push-up position, hold for a beat and then walk back to the standing position.
- Pick up the ball and repeat for the designated repetitions or time.

Key Performance Points

- Brace the core strongly to prevent the ribs and hips from being separated during the slam.
- Step to the side instead of being over the top of the medicine ball if needed.

RIP TRAINER LOW SLAP SHOT

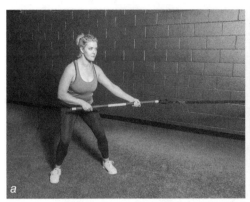 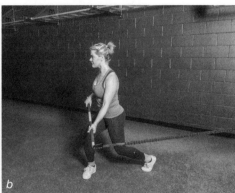

Setup and Performance

- Anchor a "rip stick" cord to a solid attachment that is at about hip height. Hold the rip stick with an underhand grip on the top hand and an overhand grip on the bottom hand.
- Turn sideways to the attachment point and move out until the cord has tension.
- Set the feet a bit wider than shoulder-width apart and the hips pushed back slightly holding the stick with both hands across the body.
- Sit back and slightly down while turning the shoulders perpendicular to the hips.
- Strongly drive the floor away while rotating open, and swing the stick to about knee height at the finish.
- Repeat for the designated time or repetitions.

Key Performance Points

- Perform these with a high cadence. They should be done rapidly and powerfully.
- Allow the back foot to pivot on the follow-through.

MEDICINE BALL CROSS-BEHIND SIDE SCOOP THROW

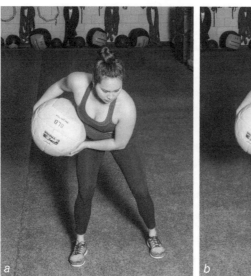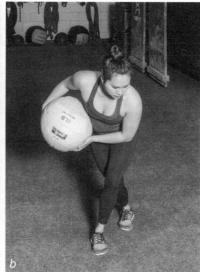

Setup and Performance

- Holding a medicine ball in the hands, turn sideways to the wall and about 10 feet (3 m) back from it.
- Set the feet a bit wider than shoulder-width apart with the hips pushed back, holding the ball with both hands across the body.
- Perform a cross-behind step (stepping toward the wall) with the foot furthest from the wall. Step back out toward the wall with the other foot.
- Simultaneously, sit back and slightly down while turning the shoulders perpendicular to the hips.
- Strongly drive the floor away while rotating open, and throw the ball into the wall explosively, turning the hips at the wall on the follow-through.
- Catch the ball, reset, and repeat.

Key Performance Points

- Throw the ball hard; try to "break" the ball.
- Sit into the hips to properly load them for the throw. The hips are the motor.
- Scoop the ball with both hands as it is thrown at the wall.

SUSPENSION TRAINER SQUAT HANG BREATHING DRILL

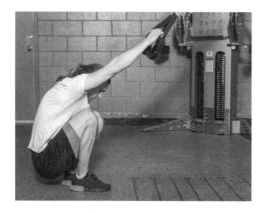

Setup and Performance

- Set the suspension trainer straps to the fully lengthened position.
- Sit down into the bottom of a natural squat with the butt as close to the heels as possible and the arms up holding the suspension trainer straps.
- The arms should be straight and the feet as close together as possible with the right foot a couple of inches in front of the left foot.
- Breathe in through the nose and out through the mouth feeling the ribs press against the thighs and the low back filling up with air for the designated amount of breaths.

Key Performance Points

- This is actually not a squat, per se, and it is not loaded so it has different guidelines. The purpose of this exercise to restore the body to a more parasympathetic state after training.
- The lumbar spine will be slightly rounded in this exercise to get the body back out of excessive lumbar extension and back to a more neutral state.

SUSPENSION TRAINER BODY SAW

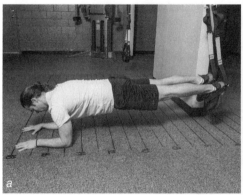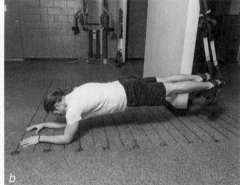

Setup and Performance

- Set the suspension trainer with the bottom of the foot straps measuring to about midshin. Place the feet in straps so that they are even when facing the ground.
- Get into a front plank position with the elbows stacked directly under the shoulder joints, and the forearms parallel to each other.
- Maintain the plank position while pushing the body away from the shoulders. Pull back into the starting position with the shoulders stacked over the elbows or very slightly in front of them.

Key Performance Points

- Keep the face pushed away from the ground and the neck in a neutral position.
- This is an exercise that should not be felt in the lumbar spine
- Keep full body tension while moving forward and backward to maintain the core cannister position.

FLOOR LADDER FORWARD WIDE-OUT

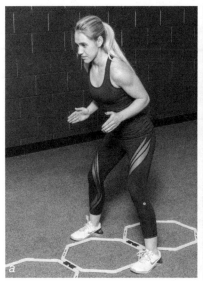
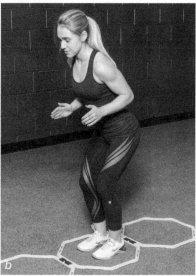

Setup and Performance

- Stand with both feet outside and straddling the first rung of the ladder.
- Jump both feet into the first rung and then back out moving forward toward the next rung.
- Continue moving up the length of the ladder at the appropriate speed.

Key Performance Point

Perform the pattern slowly at first and then work to move faster and faster.

SANDBAG COMPLEX: HIGH PULL, BENT-OVER ROW, PUSH PRESS, ALTERNATING LATERAL-STEP ROMANIAN DEADLIFT–CLEAN

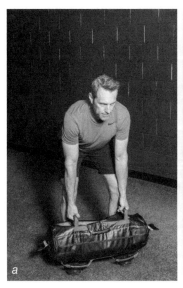
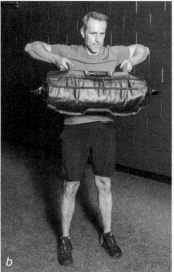
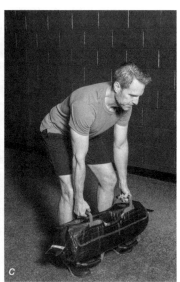

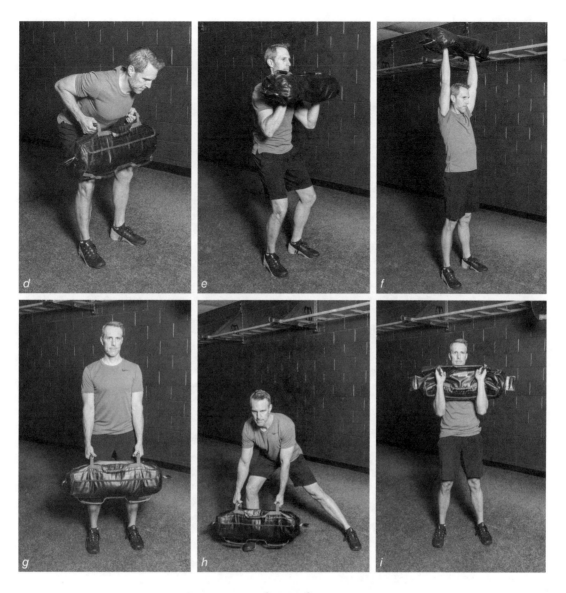

Setup and Performance

- Stand with feet about hip-width apart holding a sandbag in front of the body with the arms straight and hands holding the neutral-grip handles.
- Set up in a deadlift starting position with the bag on top of the feet. Perform a high pull by pushing the floor away and "floating" the bag with the impulse from the hips. The elbows will be above the bag and the bag will end at midchest height. Perform all the reps of the high pull.
- Bend at the hips while keeping the spine neutral, and perform the designated repetitions of the bent-over row.
- After completing the bent-over row repetitions, perform one clean so that the bag lands on top of the fists.
- Perform a sandbag push press for the designated repetitions.
- Bring the bag back down and perform alternating lateral-step Romanian deadlift and cleans (as previously described) for the designated repetitions.

Key Performance Points

- The torso should be almost horizontal to the floor on the bent-over rows.
- Keep the sandbag close to the body on the high pulls and ensure that it is hip-powered not arm-powered. The arm only serves as a guide.
- End with the sandbag directly above the crown of the head on the push press.

MEDICINE BALL FRONT SQUAT + FLOOR SLAM

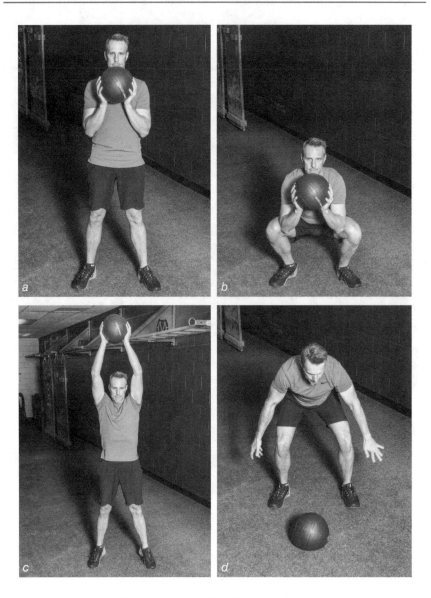

Setup and Performance

- Hold a medicine ball (ideally a nonbouncing medicine ball) in front of the body in the goblet position.
- Set the feet about shoulder-width apart with the toes turned out slightly. Stand tall.
- Squat down between the feet so that tops of the thighs are below parallel to the floor.
- Come back to the top and bring the ball overhead. Slam the ball down on the ground just in front of the feet.
- Pick up the ball and repeat for the designated repetitions or time.

Key Performance Points

- Be sure the knees track in line with the toes.
- Maintain the depth standard on the squats as fatigue accumulates.

SANDBAG BIRDDOG LATERAL DRAG

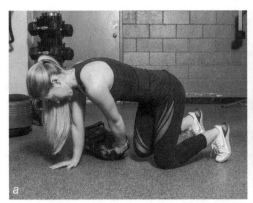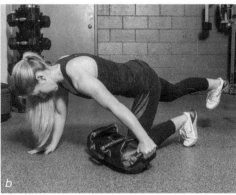

Setup and Performance

- Start on the hand and knees, the knees under the hips and the hands under the shoulders. Both the hands and knees are about shoulder-width apart. The toes are tucked under.
- Grip the floor with the hands. The sandbag will start on one side of the body.
- Grab the outside handle of the sandbag with the opposite side hand (i.e., if the bag is on the left side of the body, grab it with the right hand, dragging the bag from left to right) as you pick up the knee diagonal to this hand.
- The thumb of the hand pulling the bag will point forward. As you pull the bag underneath you, extend the leg opposite to the hand dragging away from you. This will leave two points of contact on the ground and one hand on the sandbag. Once the bag is pulled as far as possible without losing position, switch the hands and legs and go back in the other direction.

Key Performance Points

- Maintain a stable pelvis while the bag is moving and the point of stability from the leg is removed.
- When the bag is being pulled, keep it low, pulling it under the stomach, just slightly in front of the belly button. It should be closer to the thighs than it is to the arms.
- Pull slowly! Keep bag even and flat on the ground as you drag.

KETTLEBELL DEAD SWING

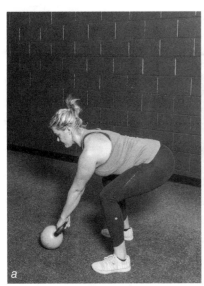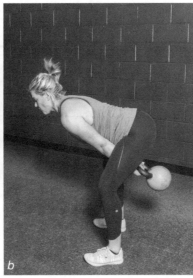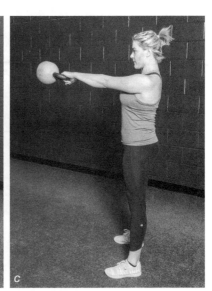

Setup and Performance

- Set the kettlebell 8 to 12 inches (20-30 cm) in front of the toes with the feet slightly wider than shoulder-width apart.
- Place both hands on the kettlebell handle, tilt the bell back so it forms a straight line with the arms.
- The body position will resemble a starting deadlift position with the hips higher than the knees but lower than the shoulders. Create full body tension prior to swinging the bell back.
- Hike the bell back, keeping the arms above the knees.
- Push the feet down into the floor and stand up straight aggressively, using the hips. The bell swings forward from the power provided from the hips to about chest level.
- Keep the hips extended while the bell starts to come downward. When the arms begin to reconnect with the ribs, push the hips back for the backswing.
- Complete the backswing and park the kettlebell back on the floor in its original position. Repeat for the designated reps.

Key Performance Points

- These swings are done one at a time. Think of each set as eight sets of one repetition rather that a single set of eight.
- Swings are hip-powered, not arm-powered. This is a key concept to teach.
- Sniff in the air on the downswing and hiss out the air when the hips extend.
- Keep the spine stable during the swing and the arms straight.
- The body should look like a perfect plank at the top position.

WALL 90/90 BREATHING DRILL

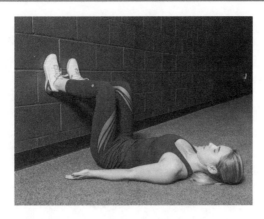

Setup and Performance

- Lie down on the floor with the feet on the wall, with the hips and knees both flexed to 90-degree angles with the arms at the sides.
- Breathe in through the nose and fully exhale out through the mouth for the designated amount of breaths.

Key Performance Points

- Think of starting the breath low. Start the breath in the feet and fill up from there.
- Breath in circumferentially (360-degree expansion), not just into the "belly," but all the way around.
- The purpose of this exercise is to help restore the body to a more parasympathetic state after training.
- The feet are on the wall to help facilitate a slightly posteriorly tilted pelvis.
- Repeat for the designated number of breaths.

GOBLET CROSS-BEHIND LUNGE

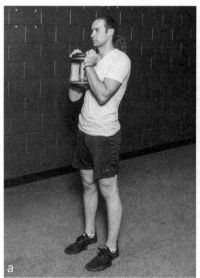
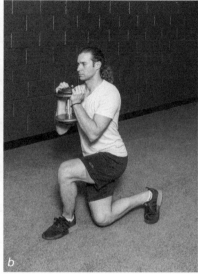

Setup and Performance

- Start by standing in a split stance holding a dumbbell or kettlebell in the goblet position in front of the chest with the feet about hip-width apart.
- Step back with one leg diagonally behind the front leg.
- Sit back and down so that the rear knee almost touches the ground.
- Push through the front foot and return to the starting position. Repeat.

Key Performance Points

- Keep the hips squared to the front.
- Before loading this movement, make sure that you are stepping the correct distance back and across by checking if the knee of the back leg drops to the outside and just behind the heel of the stationary leg.

SANDBAG COMPLEX: STAGGERED-STANCE BENT-OVER ROW AND CLEAN + PUSH PRESS

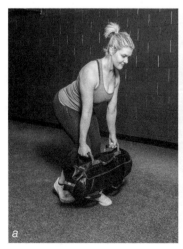
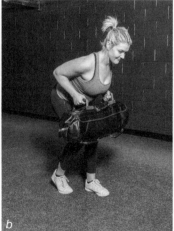
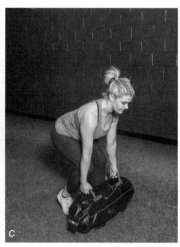

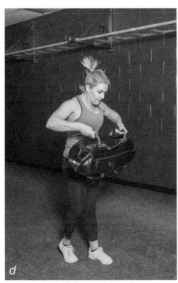 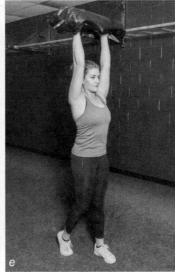 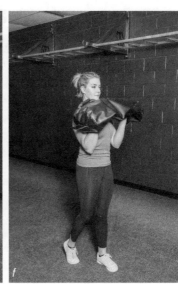

Setup and Performance

- Stand with the feet hip-width apart and slide one foot back so the toe of the back foot is in line with the heel of the front foot or up to a few inches behind it. Hold the sandbag in front of the body with the arms straight and the hands holding the neutral-grip handles.
- Keep the back heel elevated off the floor, with most of the weight in the front foot. (The back foot serves primarily as a kickstand.)
- Bend at the hips and perform the designated number of bent-over row repetitions with the feet in the staggered-stance position.
- After completing the bent-over row repetitions, stand and perform a sandbag clean so that the bag lands on top of the fists. From this position, immediately perform a push press with the feet in the staggered-stance position. Perform the designated number of repetitions.
- Next, switch the stance with the feet and repeat the process on the other side.

Key Performance Points

- The torso should be almost horizontal to the floor on the bent-over rows.
- Keep the sandbag close to the body on the cleans and ensure that it is hip-powered not arm-powered. The arm only serves as a guide.
- Complete the exercise with the sandbag directly above the crown of the head on the push press.

SANDBAG ALTERNATING FRONT AND REVERSE LUNGE UP-DOWN

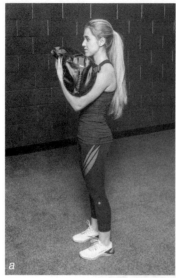
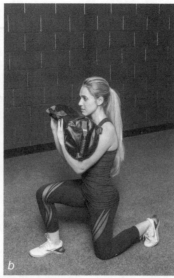
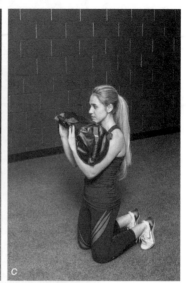

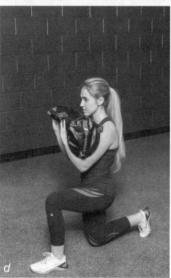
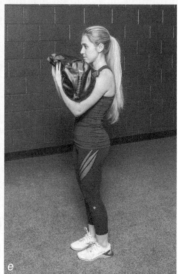

Setup and Performance

- Stand with the feet about hip-width apart holding a sandbag in front of the body in the crooks of the elbows.
- Step back with one foot and drop into a reverse lunge position, but put the back knee on the ground under the hip into a half-kneeling position.
- Stay tall and bring the front knee slightly around and back into a tall-kneeling position.
- Next, bring the leg that originally stepped backward at the beginning to the front into a half-kneeling position on the other side.
- Push through both feet back to the top position and repeat this process starting with the opposite leg.

Key Performance Points

- Pull the bag in toward the body with the arms to connect the upper and lower body together.
- Keep the torso relatively vertical.
- Keep the eyes forward.

CHAPTER 9

The Fitness Coach's Toolbox of Workouts

In the fitness industry, we have become quite enamored with tools. Alwyn often tells the story that when the suspension trainer first came out, we didn't want to purchase any because it would add a big expense to the gym. But in the end, we were compelled to buy them because they were a unique and superior way of performing certain exercises. The instability component of the suspension trainer came from the top-down versus the bottom-up, which was something that we didn't get with other tools. We realized that we couldn't afford to be without them because of their superiority and versatility.

When a new tool comes on the scene, these are the first questions we ask must ask ourselves:

- How does this tool improve on the tool we are currently using?
- What makes this tool unique compared to something else?
- Does this tool fit within our preexisting training system and training principles?

The last question is key; when we use a tool, we want to make sure it is a match for our programming system. Rather than just having a bunch of stuff, we want to make sure the tool is a fit for us. We integrate the tool into our preexisting system rather than choosing a tool and then building the system around it. A system that is based on principles comes first, and the addition of any tools comes after this has been established. Basing the system on principles makes choosing tools much easier because they can be filtered based on their utility.

Alwyn has stated that we should look at fitness training similar to how an MMA (mixed martial arts) school views combat training. We use an integrated training approach, especially in terms of our tools and methods. Just as an MMA school wouldn't teach only kickboxing, striking, or jujitsu, we don't teach only sandbag, suspension trainer, barbell, dumbbell, or kettlebell classes. Instead, we have classes and programs that are based on thematic goals such as fat loss or strength. The tools that we choose best accomplish our objectives and goals for the client and for the class. This is not to say that we can't instruct a class or design a training session to teach or utilize just one specific tool if we have limits imposed on us. We can and will do this at times. But once again, we first determine the goal and then decide which tools will best help us accomplish that goal or task at hand. What we don't want to do is to try to use a hammer when we need a screwdriver. We have a fully equipped gym, and our training sessions simply combine the use of various essential tools, so we are rarely forced to have equipment or tool constraints imposed upon us.

If you remember back to the very start of the book, we stated that "we write programs, not just workouts." Thus far, this book has been all about the process of designing programs, but sometimes a workout is needed that was not part of the original plan. The situation may arise when you may be forced to call an audible and deviate from an intended plan. Even in this situation, it starts by determining the intended objective or purpose of the session. Think of it as a minigoal for the day.

When someone needs to perform a workout for a particular reason, we usually suggest using a piece of one of the other plans in this book based on the client goal and training age, but there are some unique situations that need to be addressed differently. We can predesign some training sessions to use when these unique situations arise. The training formats will not look that different from the plans you have previously seen, but we will manipulate the exercise selection quite a bit due to the client's logistical constraints. That context is critical to understanding the programs presented in the upcoming training sessions.

At the hundreds of seminars we have attended over the years, the question that many presenters get asked (and tend to dread) is, "If you could only do one exercise, what would it be?" Context is always king, and this is why experts often give the equally dreaded answer of "it depends." It *always* depends!

Gray Cook has stated, "Everyone is looking for absolutes, when there is only context and relativity." This has always stuck with us; the more you learn the more you realize that "it depends" is one of life's truths. The problem with "it depends" is if that is where it is left. You have to follow up with what it depends upon. The follow-up from the presenter being asked the question about their one favorite exercise is almost always, "For what purpose and for whom?" Specifics matter.

The reality is that you almost never have to choose only one exercise or get to that extreme level of minimalism in most situations, so the point is kind of moot. That said, you may have several other constraints and may need to construct an effective training session within a given scenario.

You may have to design a program around these client constraints (notice that some of the constraints involve the use of one type of tool):

- Bodyweight only
- Dumbbell only
- Barbell only
- Vacation or travel
- New prospective client
- Lower-body only
- Upper-body only
- Core conditioning

The difficult part in providing various preplanned implement- or constraint-based training sessions is scaling the training sessions up or down to fit the client in front of you. This is where the exercise progression and regression principles you learned earlier will be put to use.

As much as possible, we want each training session to be related to the client goal. This must be considered for the training to have purpose. That said, the following training sessions will have the general goal of strength and hypertrophy to make it applicable for a wide range of clients. Therefore, the strength and hypertrophy rep ranges are used throughout the training sessions listed.

Bodyweight-Only Workout

Almost a decade ago, Alwyn wrote an article titled, "Your Body Is a Barbell: No Dumbbells, No Barbells, No Problem" (Cosgrove 2011). The article states that "As far as a fitness enthusiast is concerned, muscle tension comes when you place resistance on the muscles. It doesn't matter what form the resistance takes. As far as the muscles are concerned, resistance is resistance. The muscles have no idea what form the resistance takes, whether it is dumbbell, a resistance band, a barbell, or your bodyweight."

To a body, it's all resistance training; the desired training effects still follow, and we use the same guidelines mentioned previously. Many people are of the mistaken idea that one can't get strong from using bodyweight-only training. This couldn't be further from the truth. There exists a myriad of ways to get strong using bodyweight training and, in fact, we regularly include some form of bodyweight training in almost all of our complete training plans. On certain movements, some clients may hit a ceiling in which their bodyweight is not enough to make them stronger or bigger. At that point they will need to externally load the movement, but we can also manipulate body positions, tempos (purposely slower eccentric pauses, and concentric actions), and use single-limb exercises to make bodyweight exercises quite challenging.

On a programming level, we prefer clients to become very adept at controlling their own bodyweight on a basic movement before starting to utilize the addition of loaded implements on a large scale. In other words, we generally want to see bodyweight competency in the fundamental movement patterns (and the subcategories) of push, pull, squat, and hinge before we start adding external load. Generally, if a client's exercise form looks poor without external loading, it will not improve with the addition of load.

A bodyweight-only session can be utilized for a variety of reasons, including the following:

- Lack of equipment availability (maybe the gym is ultrabusy at a certain time).
- A need to back off or deload from barbell or dumbbell work. Bodyweight work can be somewhat less systemically demanding on the body.
- Travel and lack of equipment. The accessibility of performing bodyweight training is what can also make it so useful at certain times.

Designing a single session can be as simple as performing a squat, a hinge, a push, and a pull to complete a well-rounded session. If you have determined that a bodyweight-only session is in order for a client, table 9.1 is a workout that can be used to show the utility of bodyweight-only training (the tempo key is on page 29).

Table 9.1 Bodyweight-Only Workout

			Sets	Reps	Tempo	Rest
	1.	Single-arm and single-leg tall plank	2-3	1 each side	10-15 sec	60 sec
Combina-tion or power development			Sets	Reps	Tempo	Rest
	2.	Prisoner vertical jump (reset each rep)	3-4	5	X	45 sec
Resistance training			Sets	Reps	Tempo	Rest
	3a.	Single-leg squat to box	3	6 each side	—	60 sec
	3b.	Chin-up	3	As many as possible	Mod	60 sec
	4a.	Single-leg shoulder-elevated hip bridge	3	As many as possible	Slow	60 sec
	4b.	Dip	3	As many as possible	—	60 sec
	5a.	Bent-over overhand-grip row + leg raise	2	6-8	1-5-1	N/A
	5b.	T-push-up	2	8 each side	—	60 sec

Notes:

This workout is created with the assumption that you have access to a dip station and a pull-up bar. If not, adjustments will have to be made and you will have to replace the pull and push.

The six reps on exercise 3a should be challenging. If 6 reps is not challenging you can manipulate the following:
• *Tempo*: Add a one- to five-second pause at the bottom to increase intensiveness; slow down the eccentric portion and lower over three to five seconds; or go intentionally slower on the concentric, up to three seconds.
• *Range of Motion*: Increase the range of motion and squat to a lower box or perform the squat while standing on a box. If the six reps are too challenging, increase the height of the box to decrease the range of motion.
• When we prescribe as many reps as possible (amrap), we want clients to feel like they couldn't do another rep. We are not prescribing that they get to the point in which they purposely miss a rep, but it may happen when they attempt a rep they thought they could make. If clients find that they can do more than 15 reps to standard on an amrap set, they need to increase the intensiveness by manipulating the tempo. Conversely, if they can't do at least five to six reps, they need to reduce the load of the body with a band or regress the exercise appropriately.

Dumbbell-Only Workout

Rarely have we been restricted to a dumbbell-only training session, but you may find yourself hamstrung and only have access to dumbbells because of a lack of equipment availability. Note that in designing the session in table 9.2, we have assumed that you have access to a full choice of dumbbell weights and not just a selected few.

Barbell-Only Workout

The barbell is one of our primary tools for building maximal strength. It's designed for easy incremental loading making it simple to apply the principle of progressive overload. It is also a great tool for building hypertrophy because the loads can place a high level of mechanical tension on the involved musculature.

As stated earlier, the training sessions at our gym combine the use of various tools and modalities, but if we decided that we wanted to build a session exclusively around the use of the barbell, table 9.3 shows what that can look like.

Table 9.2   Dumbbell-Only Workout

Core training			Sets	Reps	Tempo	Rest
	1.	Dumbbell tall-plank alternating row	2-3	6-8 each side	—	60 sec
Combination or power development			Sets	Reps	Tempo	Rest
	2.	Dumbbell single-arm hang power snatch	3-4	3 each side	—	60 sec
Resistance training			Sets	Reps	Tempo	Rest
	3a.	Dumbbell goblet three-second halting squat	3	8-10	—	60 sec
	3b.	Dumbbell three-point neutral-grip row	3	8-10 each side	—	60 sec
	4a.	One-dumbbell single-leg Romanian deadlift (contra)	3	10 each side	—	60 sec
	4b.	Dumbbell low-incline alternating press (alternate from top)	3	8-10 each side	—	60 sec

Notes:

Hex dumbbells work best for exercise 1 if they are available.

If the client is unable to go overhead on exercise 2, perform a dumbbell jump shrug as a substitute.

A "halting" squat is a pause on the concentric (lifting portion) in the sticking point of the exercise. For most people, this is about one to two inches (3-5 cm) above the top of the thighs parallel position in the squat.

We consider low incline to be 20 degrees, but any incline of 45 degrees or less will work.

Table 9.3   Barbell-Only Workout

Core training			Sets	Reps	Tempo	Rest
	1.	Barbell roll-out	2	6-8	Slow	60 sec
Combination or power development			Sets	Reps	Tempo	Rest
	2.	Barbell hang jump shrug	3	5	X	60 sec
Resistance training			Sets	Reps	Tempo	Rest
	3a.	Front squat	3	6	—	90 sec
	3b.	Barbell overhead press	3	6	—	90 sec
	4a.	Barbell inverted row	3	8	—	90 sec
	4b.	Barbell single-leg Romanian deadlift	3	8 each side	Mod	90 sec

Notes:

The barbell roll-out is performed like the wheel kneeling roll-out, but 25-pound (11 kg) plates are placed on the end of a barbell if a wheel is not available.

For a complete total body training session, we make sure that we squat, hinge, push, and pull in this workout.

Front squats are chosen over back squats (unless the clients are powerlifters, or they are built for back squatting) because front squats tend to be easier to teach and harder to perform incorrectly compared to the back squat.

The overhead press is our preferred barbell pushing movement when compared to the bench press. We love the fact that it is a standing plank and that there is a tremendous amount of muscle mass involved over a large range of motion. Successfully lifting weights overhead makes us happy in general!

Vacation or Travel Workout

Vacation workouts can be very difficult to design if you overthink and overcomplicate them. You always have to consider the person in front of you when you assign it. Most of the time, for a one- or two-week vacation session, we try to slightly adjust the exercises in the client's current training phase to keep the most continuity. If that is not possible, we keep the travel sessions fairly straightforward and simple so that the sessions can be easily applied.

In reality, most vacations last about one to two weeks and occur one to two times per year for most people. For clients that are consistent, they fear missing training sessions and regressing while they are on vacation, but if they have been steady and conscientious with their normal training, these vacations can serve as regeneration and recovery from intense training. They often come back refreshed and ready to resume training afterward, and the time off can serve as a deload, mentally and physically. It's fine to train without structure while on vacation; you can actually be on vacation if your training consistency warrants it. If you take a lot of vacations or travel a lot, then that's a different story. That said, if we determine that someone needs a vacation or a travel training session we need to ask the following questions:

- Will you have equipment or gym access?
- How long will you be traveling or on vacation?
- How much time will you have available to train?

We can adjust the client's current training program by simply providing them with alternatives to the exercises they currently perform. For example, if the client performs a pulldown variation at the gym, we can substitute a dumbbell row or another pulling exercise that will be available to them.

If clients don't know if they will have a gym available, or don't know how equipped it will be, one of the best things they can travel with is a pair of suspension training straps and some bands (these allow for the all-important pull pattern to be addressed adequately). If absolutely no equipment is available, then a bodyweight training session is in order, which can make the pull pattern hard to address. Table 9.4 shows what a typical travel or vacation workout may look like.

Prospective Client Workout

Surprise trial training sessions for potential clients are a very interesting and often challenging situation. They are effectively a try-out. The goal of these sessions is to impress clients without completely crushing them or making them so sore that they can't come back for a week, or so beaten that they never want to come back. The secret is to quickly and correctly estimate the best and most effective dose for the person in front of you.

At our gym, we don't jump into training someone without first performing a strategy session, but we know this is not always the case at a lot of commercial facilities. We like to know what clients are looking for, determine their goals, and get to know them a bit. If for some wild reason, we didn't have that information up front, and we just jumped into a training session on the fly, we would ask the following simple questions prior to starting the session:

Table 9.4 Vacation or Travel Workout

Core training			Sets	Reps	Tempo	Rest
	1a.	Front plank to tall plank	2	6-10	—	N/A
	1b.	Alternating side plank	2	4 each side	1-3-1	60 sec
Combination or power development			**Sets**	**Reps**	**Tempo**	**Rest**
	2.	Kettlebell swing or prisoner vertical jump	3	5	X	30 sec
Resistance training			**Sets**	**Reps**	**Tempo**	**Rest**
	3a.	Goblet tempo squat	3	8-10	3-1-3	60 sec
	3b.	One-dumbbell hand- supported single-leg neutral-grip row (contra)	3	1-12 each side	Mod	60 sec
	4a.	One-dumbbell tempo single-leg Romanian deadlift	3	8 each side	3-1-3	60 sec
	4b.	Push-up (variation of choice)	3	8-10	Mod	60 sec

Notes:

This session assumes some equipment availability such as dumbbells and a kettlebell. It also assumes that the client has proficiency in the kettlebell swing in exercise 2.

This session assumes that access to heavy dumbbells may not be a possibility, so tempo is manipulated to increase intensiveness as it was in the previous bodyweight-only program.

The push-up can, of course, be performed on an incline or with a different advanced variation. Adding a degree of autonomy in the training can help to create more buy-in and interest in the session for the client.

It is important to discuss a proper RPE with the client to make sure they are appropriately challenging themselves for the given rep targets.

This simple program is designed to be performed two to three times per week for up to one to two weeks maximum.

- What is your goal?
- When was the last time you trained intensively?
- What do you want to get out of this training session?
- Do you have any orthopedic concerns that we need to be aware of?

These four simple questions take only seconds to ask and can give you a lot of insight into guiding a safe and effective trial training session. You can't just jump in to training and expect to impress clients by how hard you can work them. You first need to show them that you care, as previously discussed. You can impress clients and show your caring by being relatable and by carefully listening to the answers they give, not by how much you can kick their butt in one session. You have to give them what you know they need, and a little of what they think they need.

Table 9.5 provides a trial training session that can be used for the general person with a goal of fat loss who you know little to nothing about. Don't be underwhelmed by its apparent simplicity. The loads can be dosed properly to make this a challenging workout.

Table 9.5   Prospective Client Workout

Core training			Sets	Reps	Tempo	Rest
	1a.	Front plank	2	1	30-45 sec	60 sec
	1b.	Cable half-kneeling anti-rotation press	2	5 each side	1-5-1	60 sec
Combination or power development			**Sets**	**Reps**	**Tempo**	**Rest**
	2.	Medicine ball floor slam	3	5	X	30 sec
Resistance training			**Sets**	**Reps**	**Tempo**	**Rest**
	3a.	Goblet squat	2-3	10-12	—	60 sec
	3b.	Suspension trainer inverted row	2-3	10-12	Mod	60 sec
	4a.	One-dumbbell slider single-leg Romanian deadlift	2-3	10 each side	—	60 sec
	4b.	Push-up	2-3	8-10	—	60 sec
Energy system training			**Sets**	**Work**	**Recovery**	
	5.	Interval	4-8	20 sec	40 sec	

Notes:

Choosing proper loads in this type of scenario is one of the true arts in coaching. Once again, it's important to ask some qualifying questions when it comes to specific exercises since you are missing the information you would typically obtain from a strategy session, such as whether or not they have done this exercise before, and if so, how long ago; or how much weight they have used, and for how many reps.

If someone has recent training experience within the past two weeks, you can approach the session with a little more aggressiveness depending on the client's expectations. If they are a true beginner, use an RPE of about five to six. The newness of the pattern at that level of effort will cause a decent amount of muscle damage at the given rep ranges.

For the beginner, make sure that you teach concisely and do not overcoach. They are there to train, and you don't want to overexplain every exercise by "verbally vomiting" everything you know. Make it brief and focus on only the most important cues.

Lower-Body-Only Workout

Having a default lower-body session at the ready is important when a client is unable to perform exercises with the upper body because of a temporary limitation or potential injury to the upper extremity (e.g., shoulder or elbow). Your client may have surprised you with this restriction and you may be in a pinch because you still want to deliver a quality training session and the client still wants to train. Should you just send the client home? If the client can't train the upper body, we still have the rest of the body to train! It's always good to be able to call an audible and have a plan B for situations such as this.

If this is the scenario with your client, look at the exercises in table 9.6 as examples and as a framework of movement patterns (an example of this is provided in chapter 11).

Upper-Body-Only Workout

What is the rationale for an upper-body-only session? Similar to the rationale for performing a lower-body-only session, the main reason would be because of the client's limitation or temporary inability to use the lower extremities. This typically comes in the form of a knee or hip issue.

Once again, think of the exercises in table 9.7 as examples or as a framework of movement patterns (another example of this is provided in chapter 11).

Table 9.6 Lower-Body-Only Workout

Core training			Sets	Reps	Tempo	Rest
	1.	Suspension trainer prone jackknife	2-3	6-10	Slow	60 sec
Combination or power development			Sets	Reps	Tempo	Rest
	2.	Box jump	3-4	5	X	60 sec
Resistance training			Sets	Reps	Tempo	Rest
	3.	Front squat	3	5	—	2-3 min (upper-extremity mobility/stability drill of choice during rest period)
	4a.	Two-dumbbell reverse lunge	3	10 each side	—	60 sec
	4b.	Swiss ball supine hip extension leg curl	3	10-12	2-1-2	60 sec

Notes:

The upper extremity is obviously used on the prone jackknife, but we are assuming that the tall plank (top of push-up position) is clear to train.

During the rest period (with a more experienced client) we will grant some autonomy and have them choose an upper extremity (UE) mobility and stability drill to perform during the rest period for active recovery.

Tempo of 2-1-2 on the Swiss ball SHELC is a two-second concentric, one-second pause after the concentric (with knees flexed), and a two-second eccentric phase.

Table 9.7 Upper-Body-Only Workout

Core training			Sets	Reps	Tempo	Rest
	1.	Hollow isometric hold	2	1	15-20 sec	60 sec
Resistance training			Sets	Reps	Tempo	Rest
	2a.	Barbell close-grip bench press	2-3	6-8	—	90 sec
	2b.	Dumbbell bench row	2-3	6-8	—	90 sec
	3a.	Dumbbell alternating overhead press	2-3	10-12 each side	—	60 sec
	3b.	Cable half-kneeling neutral-grip pulldown	2-3	10-12	—	60 sec
	4a.	Rope split-stance neutral-grip face pull	1	15-20	—	30 sec
	4b.	Cable split-stance single-arm forward press	1	15-20 each side	—	30 sec

Notes:

In this workout, a broad spectrum of rep ranges is used in one session, so we emphasize general strength with higher levels of tension, hypertrophy, and a bit of endurance and metabolic stress with the higher reps all in one session. The key is in selecting the best exercise to match the rep range.

A simple upper push and pull split was used in this training session. We started with a horizontal push and pull for exercises 2a and 2b, then a vertical push and pull for exercise 3a and 3b. This could also be inverted as an option. If we needed to stick to upper-only sessions for a longer duration than just one session, a "B" session would be set up in this fashion.

Core Conditioning Workout

We described core training earlier in chapter 3. Direct torso training is a big part of our training sessions and it is addressed regularly. We feel (and some research bears this out) that performing only compound exercises leaves some holes in our training so we fill them with direct torso training in our core section.

That stated, table 9.8 lays out a targeted core training session and, no, it's not going to be a superset of crunches and planks for an hour straight. As you may have guessed, it's going to be a session that emphasizes the core by training it with offset loads in our fundamental movement patterns. These movements change the center of mass relative to the base of support which increases the demands on core musculature to stabilize. If the goal is to train the core as a priority in a training session, these more integrated stabilization exercises will become some of our primary choices.

There is no doubt that most clients love core training. It's the ultimate way to get buy-in from a client on an exercise. All you have to say is that it's a core exercise, and— Sold! In truth, just about everything is a core exercise when you stabilize yourself in three dimensions, but we can manipulate some exercise selections to make them even more core-centric.

Table 9.8 Core Conditioning Workout

Core training			Sets	Reps	Tempo	Rest
	1a.	Kettlebell single-arm waiter's walk	2	20 yd each direction	—	0
	1b.	Suspension trainer single-leg prone jackknife	2	4-6 each side	Slow	60 sec
Combination or power development			Sets	Reps	Tempo	Rest
	2.	Kettlebell single-arm swing	3	5 each side	X	45 sec
Resistance training			Sets	Reps	Tempo	Rest
	3a.	Kettlebell single-arm front squat	3	6 each side	Mod	60 sec
	3b.	Suspension trainer single-arm inverted row	3	6 each side	Mod	60 sec
	4a.	One-dumbbell lateral lunge	3	12 each side	—	60 sec
	4b.	Dumbbell single-arm bench press on half bench	3	10-12 each side	—	60 sec

Notes:

The selected exercises require a great deal of the primary core functions mentioned in chapter 3. For example, the single-arm kettlebell swing has a strong antirotation component as does the suspension trainer single-arm inverted row.

The offset or asymmetrical loading utilized also cross-links the facial slings of the body together in many of these movements. The lats and glutes share a connection via the thoracolumbar fascia and these movements help to exploit that connection.

SELECT BODYWEIGHT-ONLY WORKOUT EXERCISES

SINGLE-ARM AND SINGLE-LEG TALL PLANK

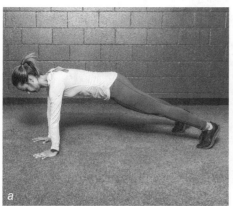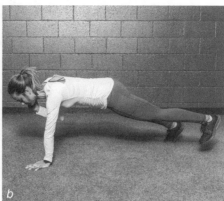

Setup and Performance

- Begin in a push-up position with the hands stacked under the shoulders and the feet shoulder-width apart or wider if needed.
- Pick up the right hand and the left foot slightly and hold the plank position.

Key Performance Points

- Shift the weight onto the two points of stability before lifting the right hand and left foot.
- Create tension by grabbing the ground with the left hand and pushing down in the ground with the right foot (switch to other side once the designated time is completed on one side).
- Keep the hips level and square while holding the plank and keep the body in a straight line. Repeat on the other side.

PRISONER VERTICAL JUMP

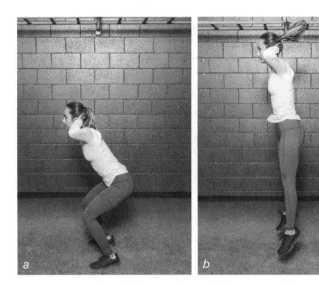

Setup and Performance

- Begin in a stance width that will allow the highest jump. Typically, this will be with the feet about hip-width apart or slightly wider.
- Interlace the fingers and place the hands behind the head in the "prisoner" position. Lower the hips down to quarter-squat depth and jump as high as possible. Land under control and reset for the next repetition.

Key Performance Points

- Commonly, this is called a squat jump but we call it a vertical jump because you don't actually perform a full squat when you attempt to jump for maximal height.
- Perform them one at a time. Treat them as doing five single reps. Reset after each jump rather than doing them continuously.

SELECT DUMBBELL-ONLY WORKOUT EXERCISES

DUMBBELL TALL-PLANK ALTERNATING ROW

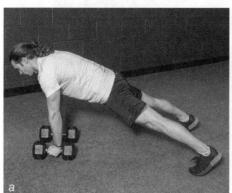 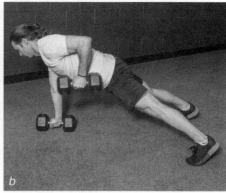

Setup and Performance

- Place two hex dumbbells on the floor. Grasp them with the hands and get into a top push-up position with the hands stacked under the shoulders and the feet shoulder-width apart or wider, if needed, to keep the hips level.
- Make sure to shift the weight (without visibly moving) onto the three points of stability, and then perform a dumbbell row with one side while maintaining a solid plank position.
- Place the dumbbells back on the ground, and alternate sides.

Key Performance Points

- This exercise is commonly referred to as a *renegade row*.
- Keep the hips level and square throughout the movement.
- Row the dumbbells toward the lower ribs rather than toward the arm pits.

DUMBBELL SINGLE-ARM HANG POWER SNATCH

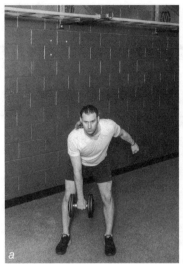 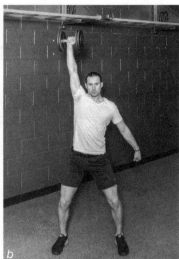

Setup and Performance

- Stand with the feet shoulder-width apart and a dumbbell in one hand.
- Push the hips back, moving into a "hang" position with the dumbbell around knee level or a bit lower and the shoulders fairly square when viewed from the front.
- Drive the floor away to explosively push the dumbbell up overhead and lock out with a fully extended arm by getting under the weight.
- The knees will be slightly bent in an athletic position when in the catch position at the top.
- Lower the dumbbell and repeat.

Key Performance Points

- Keep the dumbbell close to the body as it comes up and when returning it back down.
- This movement is hip-driven not arm-driven. Attempt to make the dumbbell "float" as much as possible by powering from the hip and pushing the feet into the floor.

SELECT BARBELL-ONLY WORKOUT EXERCISES

BARBELL ROLL-OUT

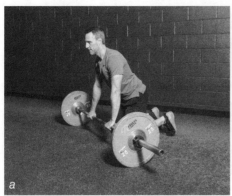 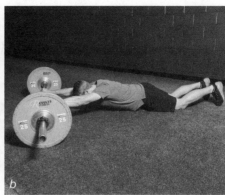

Setup and Performance

- Assume a kneeling position with the hips flexed at approximately 90 degrees. The arms are straight and the hands are gripping a barbell.
- Initiate movement of the barbell by pushing the hips forward.
- Once the hips are extended, roll the bar only as far forward as can be controlled.
- Return to the starting position and repeat.

Key Performance Points

- Lead with the hips on the way out rather than leading with the hands. On the return, lead with the hands.
- The hips should be fully extended prior to the hands moving in front of the shoulders.
- Make sure the lumbar spine does not hyperextend. The distance between the bottom of the rib cage and the pelvis stays the same as the hips move forward and the arms move out in front of the body. Keep the buttons and belt buckle (the ribs and hips) together to maintain the core cylinder.

BARBELL HANG JUMP SHRUG

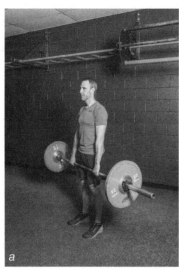 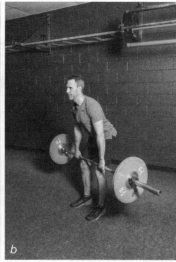 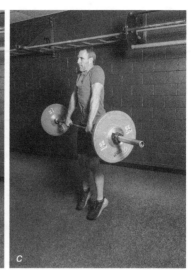

Setup and Performance

- Stand with the feet shoulder-width apart. Hold the barbell with a clean grip. This means that when you are standing with the fingers wrapped on the barbell, and you open the thumbs, they would touch the outside of the thighs.
- Push the hips back while keeping the barbell close to the legs. Lower the bar to just above the knee level.
- Reverse directions and jump while keeping straight arms and follow through by shrugging the shoulders toward the ears after the hips have extended.

Key Performance Points

- This movement is hip-driven, not arm- or shoulder-driven. Attempt to make the barbell "float" as much as possible by powering from the hip, and pushing the feet into the floor.
- Keep the barbell close to the body.
- Be sure to absorb the force of the landing by using the leg and hip as shock absorbers.

SELECT VACATION OR TRAVEL WORKOUT EXERCISES

FRONT PLANK TO TALL PLANK

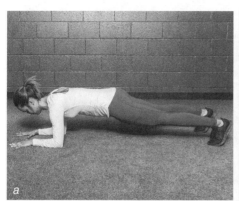 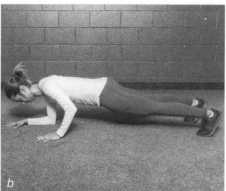

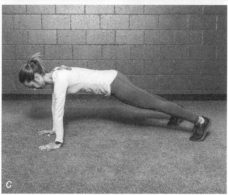

Setup and Performance

- Start on the floor in a traditional front plank position on the forearms with the palms on the ground, elbows stacked under the shoulders, and the forearms parallel to each other.
- From the front plank position, lift one forearm and place that hand on the ground and then shift the weight onto that hand. Pick up the opposite forearm and place that hand on the floor to move into a tall plank or top of push-up position.
- Reverse and go back to the front plank position.
- Repeat with the opposite arm.

Key Performance Point

- Keep the abs braced and the hips as stable as possible while making the level changes.

ONE-DUMBBELL HAND-SUPPORTED SINGLE-LEG NEUTRAL-GRIP ROW (CONTRA)

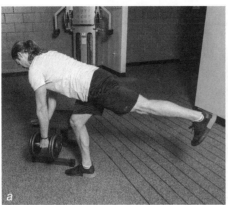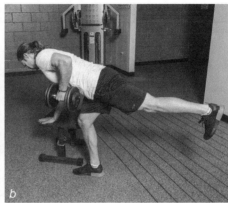

Setup and Performance

- Stand next to a bench or a box that is about 16 to 18 inches (41-46 cm) high (or higher if needed). Hinge over on the inside leg (the leg next to the bench) holding a dumbbell in the hand opposite (or contra) the stance leg.
- The back leg should be extended and straight and the body should almost form a T position. Place the free hand on the bench to provide support and keep the arm straight.
- Pull the dumbbell back toward the bottom of the ribs and slightly outside the body.
- Return to the starting position and repeat.

Key Performance Points

- When rowing, ensure that the shoulder blade is moving. A common error is to bend only the elbow without much shoulder blade movement. A good reminder for all rowing-type movement is to "spread the logo on the front of your t-shirt."
- Bring the dumbbell toward the bottom of the rib cage, not into the armpit.
- Keep the spine relatively straight and stable.

ONE-DUMBBELL SLIDER SINGLE-LEG
ROMANIAN DEADLIFT

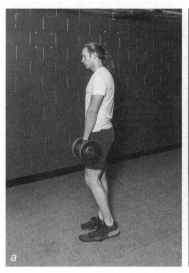 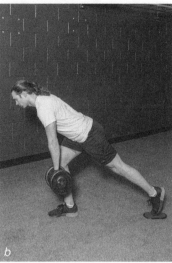

Setup and Performance

- Stand upright and place one foot, the moving leg, on a slider. The dumbbell will be on the same side as the leg that is going back.
- On the front leg you will have about a 15- to 20-degree knee bend that will allow you to push the hips to the rear. Keep the back leg pipe-straight with the forefoot on the slider.
- Keep approximately 90 percent of the weight on the nonmoving, or working, leg (the side that is doing the hip hinging).
- Hip hinge on the working leg while sliding the rear leg back.
- Push the floor away and stand upright, pulling the dumbbell up in a straight line, and repeat.

Key Performance Points

- This is an RDL. Start at the top of the lift and drive the hips mostly backward. The front shin angle will be relatively vertical.
- Keep the spine stable and move through the hips. Be sure to establish this position at the top before the lift begins.
- Be sure to keep the stance, or working leg, bent at the bottom of the movement; this is critical as it allows the hips to move back properly, if the hips don't move back you will see the hip spin open and balance will be compromised.

SELECT LOWER-BODY ONLY WORKOUT EXERCISE

BOX JUMP

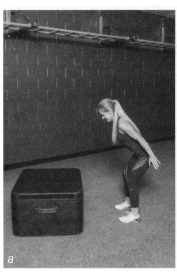 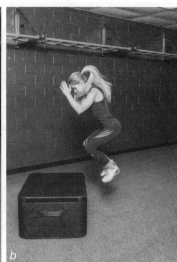 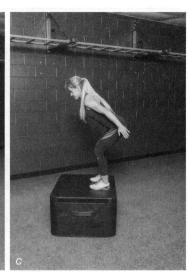

Setup and Performance

- Set up about one arm-length away from the box when in the take-off position.
- Stand tall and then dip down and jump up onto the box.
- Land in a mirror position of the take-off position, with the same amount of relative knee bend.

Key Performance Points

- A soft plyo box is recommended for this exercise.
- Keep the knees out when loading the hips on the eccentric loading for the jump.
- Land softly.
- Jump high and get maximal hip displacement.

SELECT UPPER-BODY-ONLY WORKOUT EXERCISE

CABLE SPLIT-STANCE SINGLE-ARM FORWARD PRESS

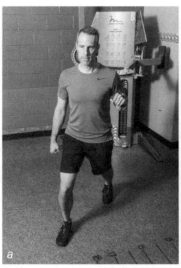 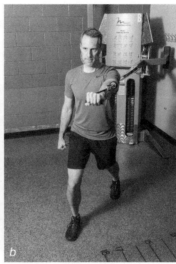

Setup and Performance

- Set a pulley to about midchest height. Grab the cable handle and split the stance into a top of split squat position.
- The hand holding the cable will be on the rear leg side or opposite the forward leg.
- Perform a single-arm press making sure to reach, allowing the scapula to protract.
- Return to the starting position under control and repeat.

Key Performance Points

- Keep the core braced and stable while pressing.
- Do not hyperextend the shoulder by allowing the elbow to travel excessively behind the torso and shoulder blade.

SELECT CORE CONDITIONING WORKOUT EXERCISE

ONE-DUMBBELL LATERAL LUNGE

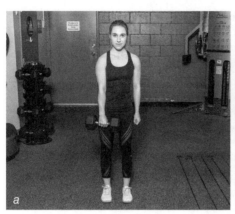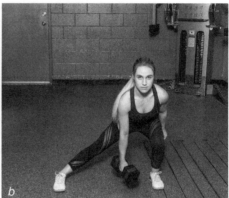

Setup and Performance

- Start with the feet together and the dumbbell held in the hand opposite the bending leg.
- Take a big step out to the side, well outside shoulder-width, and sit back and down into one side, with the trailing leg remaining straight.
- Push back into the starting position and complete the given number of reps on one side and then other.

Key Performance Points

- Keep the alignment of the ankle, knee, and hip at the bottom of the lunge. If you cut the body into an equal left and right half, and remove the trailing leg half, it would look like the bottom of a good symmetrical squat.
- Allow the torso to bend forward naturally. A common error is to try to stay overly upright on the lateral lunge.

PART III

Evaluation and Progression

CHAPTER 10

Ongoing Program Design

In chapter 1, we covered the concepts and importance of program templates. This chapter will show you how the programs in this book have been formulated. On the following pages are actual blank templates from which most of the programs were constructed. Since we showcase so many different types of full programs in this book, we had to place a limit on the number of phases that we detailed, so the programs in previous chapters are limited to two phases of programming. The following macrocycle outlines show examples of how the rep programming would progress beyond phase two.

Selecting exercises is essentially the final step in the process of designing a program. The purpose of a program template is to have about 80 percent of the work done prior to actually customizing it for a client. In this chapter's program templates, you will see that the skeleton is already in place. We then make those 20 percent tweaks based on the person in front of us. This is where the time-saving factor comes into play—you no longer have to do 100 percent of this every time you sit down to design a client program. This is the primary skill that we want you to learn and apply from this book.

One final time, let's review the four steps of program design:

1. Determine our goal.
2. Determine our starting point (training status).
3. Determine our time frame.
4. Plan backward and execute forward.

This chapter will describe step 4 in detail so that you can use these principles to successfully design your own training programs. Once again, let's take a look at figure 10.1, the illustration first shown in chapter 1 as a refresher on how the programming process for step 4 is broken down.

Select the Macrocycle Outline

Using the thought process outlined in figure 10.1, we must first select our macrocycle outline. Tables 10.1 through 10.3 are examples of the different rep programming periodization concepts used within some of our programs.

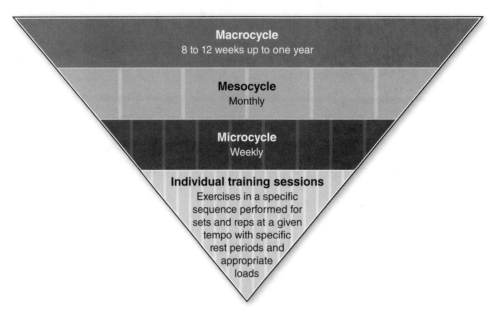

Figure 10.1   Big picture to small picture planning process.

Table 10.1   Linear Periodization Rep Programming

	Example 1	Example 2	Example 3
Phase 1	Weeks 1-4: 15 reps	Weeks 1-4: 12 reps	Weeks 1-4: 10 reps
Phase 2	Weeks 5-8: 12 reps	Weeks 5-8: 10 reps	Weeks 5-8: 8 reps
Phase 3	Weeks 9-12: 10 reps	Weeks 9-12: 8 reps	Weeks 9-12: 6 reps
Phase 4	Weeks 13-16: 8 reps	Weeks 13-16: 6 reps	Weeks 13-16: 4 reps

Table 10.2   Nonlinear Alternating Periodization Rep Programming

	Example 1	Example 2	Example 3
Phase 1	Weeks 1-4: 15 reps	Weeks 1-4: 12 reps	Weeks 1-4: 10 reps
Phase 2	Weeks 5-8: 10 reps	Weeks 5-8: 8 reps	Weeks 5-8: 6 reps
Phase 3	Weeks 9-12: 12 reps	Weeks 9-12: 10 reps	Weeks 9-12: 12 reps
Phase 4	Weeks 13-16: 8 reps	Weeks 13-16: 6 reps	Weeks 13-16: 8 reps

Table 10.3   Daily Undulating Periodization (DUP) Rep Programming

Example 1		Monday	Wednesday	Friday
Phase 1	Weeks 1-4	5 reps	15 reps	10 reps
Phase 2	Weeks 5-8	4 reps	12 reps	8 reps
Phase 3	Weeks 9-12	6 reps	20 reps	12 reps
Example 2		**Monday**	**Wednesday**	**Friday**
Phase 1	Weeks 1-4	15 reps	12 reps	10 reps
Phase 2	Weeks 5-8	12 reps	10 reps	8 reps
Phase 3	Weeks 9-12	10 reps	8 reps	6 reps

Determine the Weekly Training Split

Again, using the thought process outlined in figure 10.1, the second step, from a practical standpoint, is to determine the weekly training split within each of the phases. Tables 10.4 a-d provide some examples of different training split options for weekly sessions:

Table 10.4a Weekly Training Split: Two to Three Days per Week

Day A: full body	Day B: full body
1a. Squat (symmetrical)	1a. Hip hinge (symmetrical)
1b. Pull (horizontal)	1b. Push (vertical)
1c. Mobility/stability drill	1c. Mobility/stability drill
2a. Hip hinge (single-leg or asymmetrical)	2a. Squat (single-leg or asymmetrical)
2b. Push (horizontal)	2b. Pull (vertical)
2c. Mobility/stability drill	2c. Mobility/stability drill

Table 10.4b Weekly Training Split: Three Days per Week

Day A: squat/push/hinge/pull	Day B: push/pull/squat/pull	Day C: hinge/push/squat/pull
1a. Squat (symmetrical)	1a. Push	1a. Hip hinge (symmetrical)
1b. Push	1b. Pull	1b. Push
2a. Hip hinge (single-leg or asymmetrical)	2a. Squat (single-leg or asymmetrical)	2a. Squat (single-leg or asymmetrical)
2b. Pull	2b. Pull	2b. Pull

Table 10.04c Weekly Training Split: Three to Four Days per Week

Day A: hinge/push	Day B: squat/pull	Day C: push/hinge	Day D: pull/squat
1a. Hip hinge (primary)	1a. Squat (primary)	1a. Push (primary)	1a. Pull (primary)
1b. Push (primary)	1b. Pull (primary)	1b: Hip hinge (primary)	1b. Squat (primary)
2a. Hip hinge (secondary)	2a. Squat (secondary)	2a. Push (secondary)	2a. Pull (secondary)
2b. Push (secondary)	2b. Pull (secondary)	2b. Hip hinge (secondary)	2b. Squat (secondary)

Table 10.4d Weekly Powerlifting Training Split: Four Days per Week

Day A: lower body	Day B: upper body	Day C: lower body	Day D: upper body
1. Squat (symmetrical) "light"	1a. Push (e.g., bench press) "heavy"	1. Squat pattern (heavy)	1a. Push "light"
2. Hip hinge (symmetrical) "heavy"	1b. Mobility/stability drill	2. Hip hinge pattern (light)	1b. Mobility/stability drill
3a. Squat pattern (single-leg or asymmetrical)	2a. Push (specific assist.)	3a. Hip hinge pattern (single-leg or asymmetrical)	2a. Pull pattern (e.g. pull-up)
3b. Core	2b. Pull pattern (e.g., row)	3b. Core	2b. Push pattern (non-specific assist.)
	3. Pull (auxiliary)*		3: Pull (auxiliary)*

*Auxiliary = a tertiary exercise, often a single-joint movement, not a primary exercise.

Construct the Daily Templates

the thought process outlined in figure 10.1, the third step is to construct ramework for each training day. We need to select the number of reps, st periods for each component in our daily sessions. Once we do this, the will be selecting the specific exercise for each pattern in each component. e and power exercises are a notable exception. You will note that in the following templates, we have left the reps and tempos for those exercises blank because they are often dependent upon the exercise selected. If you preselect the reps and tempos, the exercise choices are massively restricted and often need to be changed, so we leave this section a little more open-ended. The reality is that you can pick your sets and rest periods in these components ahead of time, and then select reps and tempos after the exercises are selected.

It is worth noting that a preexisting tempo in the template may need to be adjusted after the exercise is selected so that it matches the other components. This is an outline and not set in stone, so small microadjustments are fine. As you can see, we went from big picture to small picture as we broke down this process rather than from the reverse order starting with exercises. Understanding and using this process is the key element that will help you put the *pro* in *programmer*.

Beginner to Intermediate Fat-Loss Program Templates

See tables 10.5 through 10.8 for beginner to intermediate fat-loss program templates (the tempo key is on page 29).

Table 10.5   Beginner to Intermediate Fat-Loss Program Template: Phase 1, Day A

Core training			SETS	REPS	TEMPO	REST
	1a.	Antiextension	1-2			0 sec
	1b.	Antirotation	1-2			60 sec
Resistance training			SETS	REPS	TEMPO	REST
	2a.	Squat (symmetrical)	1-3	12-15		60 sec
	2b.	Pull	1-3	12-15 each side		60 sec
	3a.	Hip hinge (single-leg or asymmetrical)	1-3	12 each side		60 sec
	3b.	Push	1-3	12		60 sec
Energy systems training			SETS	WORK	RECOVERY	
	4.	Interval	5-10	15 sec	45 sec	

Table 10.6   Beginner to Intermediate Fat-Loss Program Template: Phase 1, Day B

Core training			SETS	REPS	TEMPO	REST
	1a.	Antiextension	1-2			0 sec
	1b.	Antilateral flexion	1-2			60 sec
Resistance training			SETS	REPS	TEMPO	REST
	2a.	Hip hinge (symmetrical)	1-3	12-15		60 sec
	2b.	Push	1-3	12-15 each side		60 sec
	3a.	Squat (single-leg or asymmetrical)	1-3	12 each side		60 sec
	3b.	Pull	1-3	12-15		60 sec
Energy systems training			SETS	WORK	RECOVERY	
	4.	Interval	5-10	15 sec	45 sec	

Table 10.7   Beginner to Intermediate Fat-Loss Program Template: Phase 2, Day A

Core training			SETS	REPS	TEMPO	REST
	1a.	Antiextension	1-2			0 sec
	1b.	Antirotation	1-2			60 sec
Resistance training			SETS	REPS	TEMPO	REST
	2a.	Squat (symmetrical)	2-3	8-10		60 sec
	2b.	Pull	2-3	8-10 each side		60 sec*
	3a.	Hip hinge (single-leg or asymmetrical)	2-3	10 each side		60 sec
	3b.	Push	2-3	8-10		60 sec*
Energy systems training			SETS	WORK	RECOVERY	
	4.	Interval	5-10	20 sec	40 sec	

*During this rest period, clients will often perform a mobility and stability drill tailored to their needs and based on their FMS results, so it may be something like an active hip flexor stretch, a "rib pull" (thoracic spine rotation drill), or an ankle mobility drill.

Table 10.8   Beginner to Intermediate Fat-Loss Program Template: Phase 2, Day B

Core training			SETS	REPS	TEMPO	REST
	1a.	Antiextension	1-2			0 sec
	1b.	Antilateral flexion	1-2			60 sec
Resistance training			SETS	REPS	TEMPO	REST
	2a.	Hip hinge (symmetrical)	2-3	10		60 sec
	2b.	Push	2-3	8-10 each side		60 sec*
	3a.	Squat (single-leg or symmetrical)	2-3	10 each side		60 sec
	3b.	Pull	2-3	8-10	Mod	60 sec*
Energy systems training			SETS	WORK	RECOVERY	
	4.	Interval	5-10	20 sec	40 sec	

*During this rest period, clients will often perform a mobility and stability drill tailored to their needs and based on their FMS results, so it may be something like an active hip flexor stretch, a "rib pull" (thoracic spine rotation drill), or an ankle mobility drill.

Advanced Fat-Loss Program Templates

See tables 10.9 through 10.12 for advanced fat-loss program templates.

Table 10.9   Advanced Fat-Loss Program Template: Phase 1, Day A

Core training			SETS	REPS	TEMPO	REST
	1a.	Antiextension	2			0 sec
	1b.	Antilateral flexion	2			60 sec
Resistance training			SETS	REPS	TEMPO	REST
	2a.	Squat (symmetrical)				
		Sessions 1, 2, & 3	2-3	15		60 sec
		Sessions 4, 5, & 6	3	12		60 sec
	2b.	Pull				
		Sessions 1, 2, & 3	2-3	15 each side		60 sec*
		Sessions 4, 5, & 6	3	12 each side		60 sec*
	3a.	Hip hinge (bridge)				
		Sessions 1, 2, & 3	2-3	15		60 sec
		Sessions 4, 5, & 6	3	12		60 sec
	3b.	Push				
		Sessions 1, 2, & 3	2-3	15		60 sec*
		Sessions 4, 5, & 6	3	12		60 sec*
Energy systems training			SETS	WORK	RECOVERY	
	4.	Interval	4-7	30 sec	60 sec	

*During this rest period, clients will often perform a mobility and stability drill tailored to their needs and based on their FMS results, so it may be something like an active hip flexor stretch, a "rib pull" (thoracic spine rotation drill), or an ankle mobility drill.

Table 10.10   Advanced Fat-Loss Program Template: Phase 1, Day B

Core training			SETS	REPS	TEMPO	REST
	1a.	Antirotation	2			0 sec
	1b.	Hip flexion	2			60 sec
Resistance training			SETS	REPS	TEMPO	REST
	2a.	Hip hinge (symmetrical)				
		Sessions 1, 2, & 3	2-3	15		60 sec
		Sessions 4, 5, & 6	3	12		60 sec
	2b.	Push				
		Sessions 1, 2, & 3	2-3	12-15		60 sec*
		Sessions 4, 5, & 6	3	10-12		60 sec*
	3a.	Squat (single-leg or asymmetrical)				
		Sessions 1, 2, & 3	2-3	15 each side		60 sec
		Sessions 4, 5, & 6	3	12 each side		60 sec
	3b.	Pull				
		Sessions 1, 2, & 3	2-3	15		60 sec*
		Sessions 4, 5, & 6	3	12		60 sec*
Energy systems training			SETS	WORK	RECOVERY	
	4.	Interval	4-7	30 sec	60 sec	

*During this rest period, clients will often perform a mobility and stability drill tailored to their needs and based on their FMS results, so it may be something like an active hip flexor stretch, a "rib pull" (thoracic spine rotation drill), or an ankle mobility drill.

Table 10.11   Advanced Fat-Loss Program Template: Phase 2, Day A

Core training			SETS	REPS	TEMPO	REST
	1a.	Hip flexion	2			0 sec
	1b.	Antirotation	2			60 sec
Resistance training			SETS	REPS	TEMPO	REST
	2a.	Hip hinge (symmetrical)	2-3	10		0 sec (or as little as needed before 2b)
	2b.	Push	2-3	10		0 sec (or as little as needed before 2c)
	2c.	Squat (single-leg or asymmetrical)	2-3	10 each side		120 sec
	3a.	Pull	2-3	10 each side		0 sec (or as little as needed before 3b)
	3b.	Combination (push)	2-3	8-10		60 sec
Energy systems training			SETS	WORK	RECOVERY	
	4.	Interval	6-10	30 sec	30 sec	

*During this rest period, clients will often perform a mobility and stability drill tailored to their needs and based on their FMS results, so it may be something like an active hip flexor stretch, a "rib pull" (thoracic spine rotation drill), or an ankle mobility drill.

Table 10.12   Advanced Fat-Loss Program Template: Phase 2, Day B

Core training			SETS	REPS	TEMPO	REST
	1a.	Antiextension	2			0 sec
	1b.	Antilateral flexion	2			60 sec
Resistance training			SETS	REPS	TEMPO	REST
	2a.	Squat (symmetrical)	2-3	10		0 sec (or as little as needed before 2b)
	2b.	Pull	2-3	5-10		0 sec (or as little as needed before 2c)
	2c.	Hip hinge (single-leg or asymmetrical)	2-3	10 each side		120 sec
	3a.	Push	2-3	10		0 sec (or as little as needed before 3b)
	3b.	Combination (pull)	2-3	10 each side		60 sec
Energy systems training			SETS	WORK	RECOVERY	
	4.	Interval	6-10	30 sec	30 sec	

Beginner to Intermediate Muscle-Building Program Templates

See tables 10.13 through 10.16 for beginner to intermediate muscle-building program templates.

Table 10.13   Beginner to Intermediate Muscle-Building Program Template: Phase 1, Day A

Core training			SETS	REPS	TEMPO	REST
	1a.	Antiextension	1-2			0 sec
	1b.	Antirotation	1-2			60 sec
Resistance training			**SETS**	**REPS**	**TEMPO**	**REST**
	2a.	Squat (symmetrical)	2-3	12-15		60 sec
	2b.	Pull	2-3	12-15 each side		60 sec
	3a.	Hip hinge (single-leg or asymmetrical)	2-3	12 each side		60 sec
	3b.	Push	2-3	12		60 sec

Table 10.14   Beginner to Intermediate Muscle-Building Program Template: Phase 1, Day B

Core training			SETS	REPS	TEMPO	REST
	1a.	Antiextension	1-2			0 sec
	1b.	Antilateral flexion	1-2			60 sec
Resistance training			**SETS**	**REPS**	**TEMPO**	**REST**
	2a.	Hip hinge (symmetrical)	2-3	12-15		60 sec
	2b.	Push	2-3	12-15 each side		60 sec
	3a.	Squat (single-leg or asymmetrical)	2-3	12 each side		60 sec
	3b.	Pull	2-3	12-15		60 sec

Table 10.15   Beginner to Intermediate Muscle-Building Program Template: Phase 2, Day A

Core training			SETS	REPS	TEMPO	REST
	1a.	Antiextension	1-2			0 sec
	1b.	Antirotation	1-2			60 sec
Resistance training			**SETS**	**REPS**	**TEMPO**	**REST**
	2.	Squat (symmetrical)	2-3	8		2 min+
	3a.	Pull	2-3	8-10		60 sec
	3b.	Hip hinge (single-leg or asymmetrical)	2-3	10 each		60 sec
	4a.	Push	2-3	8-10		60 sec
	4b.	Pull (auxiliary)*	2	10-12		60 sec

*Auxiliary = a tertiary exercise, often a single-joint movement, not a primary exercise.

Table 10.16   Beginner to Intermediate Muscle-Building Program Template: Phase 2, Day B

Core training			SETS	REPS	TEMPO	REST
	1a.	Antiextension	1-2			N/A
	1b.	Antilateral rotations	1-2			60 sec
Resistance training			SETS	REPS	TEMPO	REST
	2.	Hip hinge (symmetrical)	2-3	8		2 min +
	3a.	Pull	2-3	8-10		60 sec
	3b.	Squat (single-leg or asymmetrical	2-3	10 each side		60 sec
	4a.	Push	2-3	8-10		60 sec
	4b.	Hip hinge (bridge)	2	8-10		60 sec

Advanced Muscle-Building Program Templates

See tables 10.17 through 10.20 for advanced muscle-building program templates.

Table 10.17   Advanced Muscle-Building Program Template: Phase 1, Day A

Core training			SETS	REPS	TEMPO	REST
	1.	Antiextension	2-3			60 sec
Combination or power development			SETS	REPS	TEMPO	REST
	2.	Power	3-4			30 sec
Resistance training			SETS	REPS	TEMPO	REST
	3a.	Squat (symmetrical)				
		Sessions 1 & 4	2-3	10		60 sec
		Sessions 2 & 5	2	15		60 sec
		Sessions 3 & 6	4	5		90 sec
	3b.	Pull				
		Sessions 1 & 4	2-3	10	Mod	60 sec
		Sessions 2 & 5	2	15	Mod	60 sec
		Sessions 3 & 6	4	5	Mod	90 sec
	4a.	Hip hinge (single-leg or asymmetrical)				
		Sessions 1 & 4	2-3	10 each side		60 sec
		Sessions 2 & 5	2	15 each side		60 sec
		Sessions 3 & 6	4	5 each side		90 sec
	4b.	Push				
		Sessions 1 & 4	2-3	10		60 sec
		Sessions 2 & 5	2	15		60 sec
		Sessions 3 & 6	4	5		90 sec

Table 10.18 Advanced Muscle-Building Program Template: Phase 1, Day B

Core training			SETS	REPS	TEMPO	REST
	1.	Antilateral flexion	2-3			60 sec
Combination or power development			SETS	REPS	TEMPO	REST
	2.	Combination (rotation)	2			60 sec
Resistance training			SETS	REPS	TEMPO	REST
	3a.	Hip hinge (symmetrical)				
		Sessions 1 & 4	3-4	5		90 sec
		Sessions 2 & 5	3	10		60 sec
		Sessions 3 & 6	2	15		60 sec
	3b.	Push				
		Sessions 1 & 4	3-4	5		90 sec
		Sessions 2 & 5	3	10		60 sec
		Sessions 3 & 6	2	15		60 sec
	4a.	Squat (single-leg or asymmetrical)				
		Sessions 1 & 4	3-4	5 each side		90 sec
		Sessions 2 & 5	3	10 each side		60 sec
		Sessions 3 & 6	2	15 each side		60 sec
	4b.	Pull				
		Sessions 1 & 4	3-4	5	Mod	90 sec
		Sessions 2 & 5	3	10	Mod	60 sec
		Sessions 3 & 6	2	15	Mod	60 sec

Table 10.19 Advanced Muscle-Building Program Template: Phase 2, Day A

Core training			SETS	REPS	TEMPO	REST
	1.	Antiextension	2-3			60 sec
Combination or power development			SETS	REPS	TEMPO	REST
	2.	Power	3-4			45 sec
Resistance training			SETS	REPS	TEMPO	REST
	3a.	Squat (symmetrical)				
		Sessions 1 & 4	2-3	12		60 sec
		Sessions 2 & 5	4	4		90 sec
		Sessions 3 & 6	3	8		60 sec
	3.b	Pull				
		Sessions 1 & 4	2-3	12	Mod	60 sec
		Sessions 2 & 5	4	4	Mod	90 sec
		Sessions 3 & 6	3	8	Mod	60 sec
	4a.	Hip hinge (single-leg or asymmetrical)				
		Sessions 1 & 4	2-3	12 each side		60 sec
		Sessions 2 & 5	4	4 each side		90 sec
		Sessions 3 & 6	3	8 each side		60 sec
	4b.	Push				
		Sessions 1 & 4	2-3	12		60 sec
		Sessions 2 & 5	4	4		90 sec
		Sessions 3 & 6	3	8		60 sec

Table 10.20   Advanced Muscle-Building Program Template: Phase 2, Day B

Core training			SETS	REPS	TEMPO	REST
	1.	Antilateral flexion	2-3			60 sec
Combination or power development			**SETS**	**REPS**	**TEMPO**	**REST**
	2.	Combination	2			60 sec
Resistance training			**SETS**	**REPS**	**TEMPO**	**REST**
	3a.	Hip hinge (single-leg or asymmetrical)				
		Sessions 1 & 4	3-4	4		90 sec
		Sessions 2 & 5	3	8		60 sec
		Sessions 3 & 6	3	12		60 sec
	3b.	Push				
		Sessions 1 & 4	3-4	4		90 sec
		Sessions 2 & 5	3	8		60 sec
		Sessions 3 & 6	3	12		60 sec
	4a.	Squat (single-leg or asymmetrical)				
		Sessions 1 & 4	3-4	4 each side		90 sec
		Sessions 2 & 5	3	8 each side		60 sec
		Sessions 3 & 6	3	12 each side		60 sec
	4b.	Pull				
		Sessions 1 & 4	3-4	4		90 sec
		Sessions 2 & 5	3	8		60 sec
		Sessions 3 & 6	3	12		60 sec

Beginner to Intermediate Strength-Building Program Templates

See tables 10.21 through 10.24 for beginner to intermediate strength-building program templates.

Table 10.21   Beginner to Intermediate Strength-Building Program Template: Phase 1, Day A

Core training			SETS	REPS	TEMPO	REST
	1a.	Antiextension	1-2			0 sec
	1b.	Antirotation	1-2			60 sec
Resistance training			**SETS**	**REPS**	**TEMPO**	**REST**
	2a.	Squat (symmetrical)	2-3	8		90 sec
	2b.	Pull	2-3	8-10		90 sec
	3a.	Hip hinge (single-leg or asymmetrical)	2-3	8 each side		90 sec
	3b.	Push	2-3	8-10		90 sec

Table 10.22   Beginner to Intermediate Strength-Building Program Template: Phase 1, Day B

Core training			SETS	REPS	TEMPO	REST
	1a.	Antiextension	1-2			0 sec
	1b.	Antilateral flexion	1-2			60 sec
Resistance training			SETS	REPS	TEMPO	REST
	2a.	Hip hinge (symmetrical)	2-3	8		90 sec
	2b.	Push	2-3	8-10 each side		90 sec
	3a.	Squat (single-leg or asymmetrical)	2-3	8 each side		90 sec
	3b.	Push	2-3	8		90 sec

Table 10.23   Beginner to Intermediate Strength-Building Program Template: Phase 2, Day A

Core training			SETS	REPS	TEMPO	REST
	1a.	Antiextension	1-2			0 sec
	1b.	Antirotation	1-2			60 sec
Resistance training			SETS	REPS	TEMPO	REST
	2.	Squat (symmetrical)	2-3	6		2 min+
	3a.	Pull	2-3	6	Mod	60 sec
	3b.	Hip hinge (single-leg or asymmetrical)	2-3	6 each side		60 sec
	4a.	Push	2-3	6		60 sec
	4b.	Pull (auxiliary)*	2	10-12	Mod	60 sec

*Auxiliary = a tertiary exercise, often a single-joint movement, not a primary exercise.

Table 10.24   Beginner to Intermediate Strength-Building Program Template: Phase 2, Day B

Core training			SETS	REPS	TEMPO	REST
	1a.	Antiextension	1-2			0 sec
	1b.	Antilateral flexion	1-2			60 sec
Resistance training			SETS	REPS	TEMPO	REST
	2.	Hip hinge (symmetrical)	2-3	6		2 min +
	3a.	Push	2-3	6		60 sec
	3b.	Squat (single-leg or asymmetrical)	2-3	6 each side		60 sec
	4a.	Pull	2-3	6-8 each side	Mod	60 sec
	4b.	Hip hinge (bridge)	2	8-10		60 sec

Advanced Strength-Building Program Templates

See tables 10.25 through 10.32 for advanced strength-building program templates.

Table 10.25   Advanced Strength-Building Program Template: Phase 1, Day A

Core training			SETS	REPS	TEMPO	REST
	1.	Antiextension	2-3			60 sec
Resistance training			SETS	REPS	TEMPO	REST
	2a.	Squat (symmetrical)	3-4	5		90 sec
	2b.	Pull	3-4	4-7		90 sec
	3a.	Pull	2-3	12 each side		60 sec
	3b.	Squat (single-leg or asymmetrical)	2-3	10 each side		60 sec

Table 10.26   Advanced Strength-Building Program Template: Phase 1, Day B

Core training			SETS	REPS	TEMPO	REST
	1.	Antilateral flexion	2-3			45 sec
Resistance training			SETS	REPS	TEMPO	REST
	2a.	Hip hinge (single-leg or asymmetrical)	3-4	6 each side		90 sec
	2b.	Push	3-4	5		90 sec
	3a.	Hip hinge (bridge)	2-3	10	Slow	60 sec
	3b.	Push	2-3	8-10 each side		60 sec

Table 10.27   Advanced Strength-Building Program Template: Phase 1, Day C

Core training			SETS	REPS	TEMPO	REST
	1.	Antiextension	2-3			45 sec
Resistance training			SETS	REPS	TEMPO	REST
	2a.	Squat (single-leg or asymmetrical)	3-4	6 each side		90 sec
	2b.	Pull	3-4	8		90 sec
	3a.	Squat (single-leg or asymmetrical)	2	10 each side		60 sec
	3b.	Pull	2	8-10 each side		60 sec

Table 10.28   Advanced Strength-Building Program Template: Phase 1, Day D

Core training			SETS	REPS	TEMPO	REST
	1.	Antirotation	2-3			45 sec
Resistance training			SETS	REPS	TEMPO	REST
	2a.	Hip hinge (symmetrical)	3-4	5		90 sec
	2b.	Push	3-4	5		90 sec
	3a.	Hip hinge (bridge)	2-3	10-15 each side	Slow	60 sec
	3b.	Push	2	10-15		60 sec

Table 10.29 Advanced Strength-Building Program Template: Phase 2, Day A

Core training			SETS	REPS	TEMPO	REST
	1.	Antiextension	2-3			60 sec
Resistance training			SETS	REPS	TEMPO	REST
	2a.	Squat (symmetrical)	3-4	3		90 sec
	2b.	Pull	3-4	1, 2, 3	Mod	90 sec
	3a.	Pull	2-3	10 each side		60 sec
	3b.	Squat (single-leg or asymmetrical)	2-3	8 each side		60 sec

Table 10.30 Advanced Strength-Building Program Template: Phase 2, Day B

Core training			SETS	REPS	TEMPO	REST
	1.	Antilateral flexion	2-3			60 sec
Resistance training			SETS	REPS	TEMPO	REST
	2a.	Hip hinge (single-leg or asymmetrical)	3-4	4 each side		90 sec
	2b.	Push	3-4	3		90 sec
	3a.	Hip hinge (bridge)	2-3	8	Slow	60 sec
	3b.	Push	2-3	6-8	Mod	60 sec

Table 10.31 Advanced Strength-Building Program Template: Phase 2, Day C

Core training			SETS	REPS	TEMPO	REST
	1.	Antiextension	2-3			45 sec
Resistance training			SETS	REPS	TEMPO	REST
	2a.	Squat (single-leg or asymmetrical)	3-4	3 each side		90 sec
	2b.	Pull	3-4	6		90 sec
	3a.	Squat (single-leg or asymmetrical)	2	8 each side		60 sec
	3b.	Pull (auxiliary)*	2	6-8	Slow	60 sec

*Auxiliary = a tertiary exercise, often a single-joint movement, not a primary exercise.

Table 10.32 Advanced Strength-Building Program Template: Phase 2, Day D

Core training			SETS	REPS	TEMPO	REST
	1.	Antirotation	2-3			45 sec
Resistance training			SETS	REPS	TEMPO	REST
	2a.	Hip hinge (symmetrical)	3-4	3		90 sec
	2b.	Push	3-4	3		90 sec
	3a.	Hip hinge (bridge)	2-3	8-12 each side	Slow	60 sec
	3b.	Push	2	8-12		60 sec

Beginner to Intermediate General Fitness Program Templates

See tables 10.33 through 10.36 for beginner to intermediate general fitness program templates.

Table 10.33   Beginner to Intermediate General Fitness Program Template: Phase 1, Day A

Core training			SETS	REPS	TEMPO	REST
	1a.	Antiextension	1-2			0 sec
	1b.	Antirotation	1-2			60 sec
Combination or power development			SETS	REPS	TEMPO	REST
	2.	Power	3-4	5	X	30 sec
Resistance training			SETS	REPS	TEMPO	REST
	3a.	Squat (symmetrical)	1-2	12		60 sec
	3b.	Pull	1-2	10-12 each side		60 sec
	4a.	Hip hinge (single-leg or asymmetrical)	1-2	12 each side		60 sec
	4b.	Push	1-2	12		60 sec

Table 10.34   Beginner to Intermediate General Fitness Program Template: Phase 1, Day B

Core training			SETS	REPS	TEMPO	REST
	1a.	Antiextension	1-2			0 sec
	1b.	Antilateral flexion	1-2			60 sec
Combination or power development			SETS	REPS	TEMPO	REST
	2.	Power	3-4	5	X	30 sec
Resistance training			SETS	REPS	TEMPO	REST
	3a.	Hip hinge (symmetrical)	1-2	12		60 sec
	3b.	Push	1-2	10-12 each side		60 sec
	4a.	Squat (single-leg or asymmetrical)	1-2	12 each side		60 sec
	4b.	Pull	1-2	10-12		60 sec

Table 10.35   Beginner to Intermediate General Fitness Program Template: Phase 2, Day A

Core training			SETS	REPS	TEMPO	REST
	1a.	Antiextension	1-2			0 sec
	1b.	Antirotation	1-2			60 sec
Combination or power development			SETS	REPS	TEMPO	REST
	2.	Power	3-4	5	X	30 sec
Resistance training			SETS	REPS	TEMPO	REST
	3a.	Hip hinge (single-leg or asymmetrical)	2-3	10 each side		60 sec
	3b.	Push	2-3	8-10		60 sec
	4a.	Squat (symmetrical)	2-3	8-10		60 sec
	4b.	Pull	2-3	8-10 each side		60 sec

Table 10.36   Beginner to Intermediate General Fitness Program Template: Phase 2, Day B

Core training			SETS	REPS	TEMPO	REST
	1a.	Antiextension	1-2			0 sec
	1b.	Antilateral flexion	1-2			60 sec
Combination or power development			SETS	REPS	TEMPO	REST
	2.	Power	2-3	5 each side	X	20 sec
Resistance training			SETS	REPS	TEMPO	REST
	3a.	Squat (single-leg or asymmetrical)	2-3	10 each side		60 sec
	3b.	Pull	2-3	8-10	Mod	60 sec
	4a.	Hip hinge (symmetrical)	2-3	10		60 sec
	4b.	Push	2-3	8-10 each side		60 sec

Advanced General Fitness Program Templates

See tables 10.37 through 10.40 for advanced general fitness program templates.

Table 10.37   Advanced General Fitness Program Template: Phase 1, Day A

Core training			SETS	REPS	TEMPO	REST
	1.	Antirotation	2			60 sec
Combination or power development			SETS	REPS	TEMPO	REST
	2.	Power	3-4	10	X	45 sec
Resistance training			SETS	REPS	TEMPO	REST
	3a.	Squat	2-3	10		60 sec
	3b.	Pull	2-3	8-10	Mod	60 sec
	4a.	Hip hinge (single-leg or asymmetrical)	2-3	8-10 each side		60 sec
	4b.	Push	2-3	8-10 each side		60 sec

Table 10.38   Advanced General Fitness Program Template: Phase 1, Day B

Core training			SETS	REPS	TEMPO	REST
	1.	Antilateral flexion	2			60 sec
Combination or power development			SETS	REPS	TEMPO	REST
	2.	Power	3-4	5 each side	X	20 sec
Resistance training			SETS	REPS	TEMPO	REST
	3a.	Hip hinge (symmetrical)	2-3	10		60 sec
	3b.	Push	2-3	5 each side		60 sec
	4a.	Squat (single-leg or asymmetrical)	2-3	10 each side		60 sec
	4b.	Pull	2-3	8-10 each side		60 sec

Table 10.39   Advanced General Fitness Program Template: Phase 2, Day A

Core training			SETS	REPS	TEMPO	REST
	1.	Antilateral flexion	2			60 sec
Combination or power development			SETS	REPS	TEMPO	REST
	2.	Power	3-4	4 each side	X	20 sec
Resistance training			SETS	REPS	TEMPO	REST
	3a.	Hip hinge (single-leg or asymmetrical)	2-3	6 each side		60 sec
	3b.	Push	2-3	5-7 each side		60 sec
	4a.	Squat (single-leg or asymmetrical)	2-3	6		60 sec
	4b.	Pull	2-3	6 each side		60 sec

Table 10.40   Advanced General Fitness Program Template: Phase 2, Day B

Core training			SETS	REPS	TEMPO	REST
	1.	Antirotation	2			60 sec
Combination or power development			SETS	REPS	TEMPO	REST
	2.	Power	2-3	4 each side	X	45 sec
Resistance training			SETS	REPS	TEMPO	REST
	3a.	Squat (single-leg or asymmetrical)	2-3	6 each side		60 sec
	3b.	Pull	2-3	3-5		60 sec
	4a.	Hip hinge (symmetrical, bridge)	2-3	6-8		60 sec
	4b.	Push	2-3	6-8		60 sec

Toolbox Workout Templates

See tables 10.41 and 10.42 for toolbox workout program templates for upper-body only and lower-body only.

Table 10.41   Upper-Body-Only Workout Template

Core training			SETS	REPS	TEMPO	REST
	1.	Antiextension	2			60 sec
Resistance training			SETS	REPS	TEMPO	REST
	2a.	Push (horizontal)	2-3	6-8		90 sec
	2b.	Pull (horizontal)	2-3	6-8		90 sec
	3a.	Push (vertical)	2-3	10-12 each side		60 sec
	3b.	Pull (vertical)	2-3	10-12		60 sec
	4a.	Pull (horizontal, auxiliary*)	1	15-20		30 sec
	4b.	Push (horizontal)	1	15-20 each side		30 sec

*Auxiliary = a tertiary exercise, often a single-joint movement, not a primary exercise.

Table 10.42   Lower-Body-Only Workout Template

Core training			SETS	REPS	TEMPO	REST
	1.	Hip flexion	2-3			60 sec
Combination or power development			SETS	REPS	TEMPO	REST
	2.	Jump	3-4			60 sec
Resistance training			SETS	REPS	TEMPO	REST
	3.	Squat (symmetrical)	3	5		2-3 min (upper-extremity mobility/ stability drill of choice during rest period)
	4a.	Squat (single-leg or asymmetrical)	3	10 each side		60 sec
	4b.	Hip hinge	3	10-12		60 sec

CHAPTER 11

Tracking Results

In chapter 2, we discussed how the initial assessment of a client is a necessary second step in determining an appropriate starting point for achieving established goals (the first step is determining those goals). This chapter will give an overview and provide further insight into the process we use to continually track and assess progress throughout the client's journey with us.

First, it is important to recognize that assessments are not a one-off event that only occur at the strategy session. Training is a process that is continually assessed—at the beginning, the end, and, in effect, at every single workout. One of the main reasons for ongoing assessment is to evaluate and reorientate the training program when it is required. No matter how great the training program design, course correction is often required and adjustments need to be made to make progress.

When we begin, we determine the clients' goals, calculate their physical starting point through an initial training status assessment, and design a plan to achieve their goals. Through education and past experience, we believe this plan is the most direct route, but we still need to check in along the way to make sure we are not veering off the path or slowing down. If you are on a road trip, you need to keep an eye on your gauges to monitor the fuel tank, fluids, temperature, and tire pressure. When a dashboard light goes on, it is important to pay attention to it. Similarly, there are a number of gauges that you and your clients also need to pay attention to on their journey. They need to keep an eye on their stress levels, sleep, body fat percentage, and clothing size (meaning how their clothes are fitting). All of these gauges are good indicators as to whether they are heading in the right direction, or if they need to stop for gas and pay more attention to their recovery. Regular assessments are key to moving toward the clients' goals.

When it comes to ongoing assessment and keeping the client on track, the most important responsibilities as a coach are to ensure safety, maintain effectiveness, and facilitate communication. Let's take a closer look.

Ensure Safety

Continually assessing our clients' health, safety, and susceptibility to injury is one of our number one jobs. We need to regularly assess clients' movements, range of motion, and recovery throughout their program. While the program we design may be perfectly balanced to address any movement limitations or strength deficits that we found in their initial assessment, life happens and we still need to regularly assess if they need to spend more time recovering, doing regeneration sessions, or if they are compensating in a way that could lead to injury.

You want to always keep your eyes and ears open for anything that might be a sign of an injury down the road. With that said, you can't become paranoid that they'll get hurt, and therefore, not push them to progress and get better. By observing their movement quality and response to training, you can continue to increase their training loads and they can gain strength with minimal risk of injury. Be aware that there are times you may need to refer (as mentioned in chapter 2) a client who presents with pain to a qualified medical professional; fitness professionals are not typically trained to do rehabilitation and may be crossing a line if they attempt to do so. Obviously, best judgment must be used here as to when to refer out because not all situations require outside intervention.

Fitness professionals should be trained and should be regularly assessing muscular imbalances, faulty movement patterns, and (most importantly) the client's goals. It would be great if we could "set it and forget it" but that's not how the actual art of programming and coaching works. Many times, forces outside of our control will change the direction of the plan that was initially laid out. Let's discuss some of our regular check-ins when coaching a client.

EVERY WORKOUT

At every workout, assess the clients' movements, paying particular attention if they are compensating in their movement, if they mention pain, or if they start to guard an area that is causing pain. The sooner an issue is addressed, the more likely it won't turn into a full-blown problem. For example, you should pay attention if a client says a shoulder feels tight or neck feels stiff from sleeping funny. While these don't seem like major issues, they certainly could be if they keep getting worse. Mike Boyle has previously stated, "When you ask a client if something hurts, the answer is either yes or no. Often times they'll say, 'not really just a little tight,' which means YES."

EVERY ONE TO TWO MONTHS

Every one to two months (or even more frequently if possible), rescreen your client on any of the tests in the Functional Movement Screen (see chapter 2) below a score of 2. For example, if the client lacked shoulder mobility at the start, check to make sure it has improved. This is also important to show progress, to ensure that your programming is effective, and to guide future exercise progressions and regressions if needed.

EVERY YEAR

Every year (or sooner if the client has had time off), it's a good idea repeat the entire Functional Movement Screen to make sure something hasn't crept up that you need to address. If your programming is smart, the screen should validate it and confirm that you are maintaining or improving the client's fundamental movement quality. However, if your client is an athlete in a repetitive sport or someone who has gone from an active job to a sedentary job, for example, this lifestyle change could affect mobility and movement. The FMS doesn't take long and is a great way to audit yourself and your client.

Maintain Effectiveness

Throughout a client's program, we need to measure its effectiveness. Is it working? Is your client getting faster, leaner, more powerful and stronger? The program you lay out is based on your education, experience, and initial assessment of the client's current status and goals. The more you design programs the more you will be able to predict the results with confidence. There is never going to be a time that you shouldn't check yourself and measure the a client's progress to ensure you are on the right track. Where is your client in regard to goals? How big is the difference? If the goal included fat loss over the last year, how much fat was lost? If the goal was a strength increase, what lifts improved and by how much? If the goal was muscle increase, how many pounds of muscle was gained? Did the client achieve what he or she set out to do? Let's take a look at some of the progress indicators we use to check the effectiveness of your program.

Note that these progress indicators are specific to each individual client's goals but a few will apply to all. You may need to perform more specific tests depending on the client, but most fall under one of three categories: Look better, feel better, or perform better. Think about what you are measuring—Does the client want to look better? If so, body composition or clothes-fit will be an important measurement. If there are performance goals, then test the skills applicable to the sport being performed, such as a vertical jump test, a mile run, or a 1 rep max deadlift. If the goal is to feel better, the FMS might be an important indicator. The following are some suggestions on what metrics to track and how often to track them:

EVERY WORKOUT

Ask yourself if the client's loads are increasing and if the client is getting stronger. These are important because if the client isn't progressing, then you aren't doing your job correctly. If the client has performed a couple of workouts in a row with no increase in load or reps, it's probably time to change the program or address recovery issues.

Monitor heart rate during metabolic interval workouts, which is usually one to two times per week for most clients. First, make sure that the client's max heart rate is set properly using the max heart rate formula (220 – age) as an estimate. A client should be unable to carry on a conversation at 85 percent or so and able to recover to 70 percent or less. Heart rate also tells you a lot as a coach once you have it set properly. If a client is fatigued, you'll know because he or she will be unable to raise heart rate. This is a sign that a day off is needed to recover.

EVERY MONTH

- Track body composition once a month. We currently use a top-of-the-line bio-impedance unit at our gym for a variety of reasons: it is noninvasive, gives a reasonably accurate estimate of body fat, and is quick and easy to use. We recommend that our body transformation clients use it monthly to see trends and track change over time. The common question that is asked about all body composition measures is, "How accurate is it?" All of the various methods that test body fat are estimates, none of them are 100 percent accurate, and all of them have various pros and cons. We prefer our method because even though it doesn't tell us a person's exact body fat percentage, if we are consistent in its utilization, it does tell us if body fat is going up or down.

- Monitor weight once a month, or more often if your client is a weight-class athlete training to be at a certain weight. For the average client, however, we don't emphasize weight and instead use body composition or clothing-fit to measure progress.

- Use clothing as a benchmark. You can have your client bring in clothing that is currently too small. This takes the focus off the scale and on to building muscle and changing the body. Have the client try on these clothes every three to four weeks (for a period of 8 to 12 weeks total) to realize the transformation. Shifting focus from the scale can be healthy for the mindset, especially for women.

- Employ specific performance tests. These vary widely depending on the athlete, sport, and goals. There are multiple tests that can be used and it is beyond the scope of this book to cover them all.

Facilitate Communication

We must communicate regularly with our clients, to provide advice or the knowledge they need to progress while making sure they enjoy the process and stay consistent. We can write the perfect training program but if clients miss workouts, or personal issues start to affect training, things won't always go as planned. Thus, it is important to have a way to regularly check in and communicate with your clients to assess their readiness to train, their consistency, and their stress levels.

This time can also be used to discuss nutrition, which can make or break results. A bad diet, or one high in inflammatory foods, can often yield chronic aches and pains. As the saying goes, "We can't out-train a bad diet." Thus, establishing a way to regularly inquire about nutrition is extremely important. If you are coaching in-person, this check-in occurs more regularly; you get to know your client and can tell when something is off. Don't be afraid to ask questions, and be open to listening.

Also, what we say to our clients during their training journey can be extremely powerful, and our words will often stay with them. We have to take time to listen and say the right things to keep them moving forward. When clients first start training, they are always motivated, focused, and ready to do everything you ask of them. Your job really starts when life inevitably gets in the way, circumstances change, or obstacles arise, and they start to lose the motivation and focus to keep their original commitment. To help keep the lines of communication open, we do a formal monthly review in which we ask clients for input on their program and about what is working and what isn't (see figure 11.1).

Let's take a look at the regular communication checks that we use throughout the coaching process, which are in place to help clients reach their goals.

EVERY WORKOUT

Is the client sleeping well? How many hours does the client sleep? Check in regularly. Sleep is when our bodies repair and restore themselves.

How is the client fueling the body? Is breakfast a priority? You can often tell that a client isn't eating enough if workouts are flat and the client is unable to perform a typical workout. Also make sure the client consumes post-workout nutrition to refuel and replenish.

What is the client's appearance? Is there "facial freshness," with the client looking well-rested and healthy? If not, ask them about sleep.

Does the client seem motivated and focused, or distracted? Is the client still excited and focused to reach the established goals or is he or she losing steam? At every workout, you should discuss the client's goals, why you were hired, and try to reignite the fire.

How is the client feeling today? Figure 11.2 provides a training readiness chart we occasionally use with our clients before they start a training session.

Figure 11.1 Client feedback form.

Client name:______________________________ Date: ______________________________

1. What are your current (specific) goals: ______________________________

____

____

2. Are there any exercises/movements that you are currently doing that you would like to change? ______________________________

____

____

3. Are there any exercises/movements that you would like to be doing that you aren't currently doing? ______________________________

____

____

4. Do you have any recent specific physical issues or concerns? ______________

____

____

5. I feel like I am being pushed (circle one):

Too hard Just right Not hard enough

Please explain: ______________________________

____

____

6. Do you feel like you are making progress toward your goals (circle one)?

Yes No

Please explain: ______________________________

____

____

7. How many days per week are you currently able to train? ______________

8. Is there anything we can help with? ______________________________

____

____

From A. Cosgrove and C. Rasmussen, *Secrets of Successful Program Design: A How-To Guide for Busy Fitness Professionals* (Champaign, IL: Human Kinetics, 2021).

	5	**4**	**3**	**2**	**1**	**Score**
Sleep Quality	Great!	Good	Hard to Fall Asleep	Restless Sleep	Insomnia	
General Muscle Soreness	Feeling Great!	Feeling Good	Normal	A Little Sore	Very Sore	
Stress Level	Very Relaxed	Relaxed	Normal	Feeling Stressed	Very Stressed	
Fatigue	Very Fresh	Fresh	Normal	More Tired Than Usual	Very Tired	
Mood	Very Positive!	Good Mood	Less Interested	Snappy at Times	Very Irritable	

Figure 11.2 Client training readiness.

EVERY MONTH

Is the client consistent with training? Has the client been able to come in and do all of the planned workouts for this past month? Was it too much? Could the client handle more?

Is the client healthy? Take note if he or she seems to be getting sick a lot. This is a sign of a weakened immune system. Is the client overtraining? Are there outside stressors?

EVERY YEAR

Each year when a client renews with you, spend some time reflecting on past training and planning for the year ahead. What went well this past year? What would the client like to do better? Were goals accomplished? What does the client want to accomplish the following year?

Appendix

Basic Training Cycle Process with Progression

The average client stops adapting to a program in about three to six exposures to a certain stimulus, roughly a four- to six-week time period. During this time frame, we should also progressively strive to increase the client's overload, and that often means increasing the intensity.

In our basic training cycle, each step represents a week, so although we may do an A or a B session twice in a week, we typically only make the intensity adjustments once a week unless the loads need to be adjusted or the client is very new.

Week One: Intro Week

- Typically, new exercises are introduced in this phase, so the focus is on teaching correct technique so the client can develop good form. Introduction weeks can also serve as a type of deload from the previous hard phase, allowing fatigue from the previous cycle to dissipate before the client begins a new climb.

- Submaximal loads are used for the designated rep target. The client works on a reps-in-reserve idea (basically two or three reps left in the reserve).

- A reduced set and total rep volume is used. For example, the program may call for two to three sets of each exercise. In the introductory week, the client will typically perform only two sets of each.

Week Two: Base Week

- With regard to loading, the experienced client looks to repeat previous personal bests (or come very close to), while a beginner keeps one or two reps in the tank. The client should not train to positive failure, but select manageable loads for the rep target.

- Increase weight on two to three of the main exercises (not all of them).

- Increase the number of sets to the prescribed number.

Week Three: Load Week

- The client starts to push it, in regard to loading, and looks to set a new personal best in the lift (based on last week's performances).
- Increase loading on another two to three exercises.
- Full volume (sets and reps).
- Work hard. Although attempting what is essentially supramaximal work, we do not want clients to attempt a rep that they are not sure that they will be able to complete. Try to avoid technique breakdown.

Week Four: Load (PR) Week

- The client works from previous personal bests and leaves nothing in the tank this week. This is an intense week of training. The client should try to set new records.
- The client engages in full set volume, plus advanced overload techniques if necessary (e.g., drop set, forced reps).
- Minimize technique breakdown; however, the client may miss a rep or a lift at this stage. (This should only ever occur at this stage, and going to failure as a goal is not recommended.)

Week Five: New Program

- The same rules apply as week one. The client backs off on the loading and set volume, but usually works from a higher loading perspective.
- New rep ranges or exercises are usually introduced at this point.
- Using this model, we integrate the client's recovery into the intro weeks and the progression in volume and loading without risk of overtraining.

References

Chapter 1

Carroll, L., H. Haughton, and L. Carroll, L. 2009. *Alice's adventures in Wonderland; and, Through the looking-glass and what Alice found there*. New York: Penguin Classics.

Chapter 2

Burton, L., and G. Cook. 2015. Functional Movement Systems FMS Level One Manual. https://www.functionalmovement.com/Store/35/fms_level_1_online_course.

Cook, G., M. Bryan, L. Burton, K. Kiesel, and G. Rose. 2010. *Movement*. Aptos, CA: On Target Publications.

Faigenbaum, A., and R. Lloyd. 2016. "Age- and Sex-Related Differences and Their Implications for Resistance Exercise." In *Essentials of Strength Training and Conditioning*, 4th ed., edited by Greg Haff and Travis Triplett, 136-137. Champaign, IL: Human Kinetics.

Schmidt, R.A. 1991. *Motor Learning and Performance: From Principles to Practice*. Champaign, IL: Human Kinetics.

Chapter 3

Bolton, A., and P. Tsatsouline. 2012. *Deadlift Dynamite*. Little Canada, MN: Dragon Door.

Boyle, M. 2016. *Functional Training for Sports*, 2nd ed. Champaign, IL: Human Kinetics.

Childs J.D., D.S. Teyhen, T.M. Benedict, J.B. Morris, A.D. Fortenberry, R.M. McQueen, J.B. Preston, A.C. Wright, J.L. Dugan, and S.Z. George. 2009. "Effects of Sit-Up Training Versus Core Stabilization Exercises on Sit-Up Performance." *Medicine and Science in Sports and Exercise* 41, 2072-83.

Cook, G., M. Bryan, L. Burton, K. Kiesel, and G. Rose. 2010. *Movement*. Aptos, CA: On Target Publications.

Escamilla, R.F., M.S. McTaggart, E.J. Fricklas, R. DeWitt, P. Kelleher, M.K. Taylor, A. Hreljac, and C.T. Moorman. 2006. "An Electromyographic Analysis of Commercial and Common Abdominal Exercises: Implications for Rehabilitation and Training." *Journal of Orthopaedic and Sports Physical Therapy* 36(2): 45-57.

Henkin, J. 2019. Dynamic Variable Resistance Training (DVRT) Level 1 Certification Manual. DVRTFitness.com. https://ultimatesandbagtraining.com/product/dvrt-level-online-certification/

McGill, Stuart. 2007. *Low Back Disorders: Evidence-Based Prevention and Rehabilitation*. Champaign, IL: Human Kinetics.

McGill, S. 2015. *Back Mechanic: The Step-by-Step McGill Method for Fixing Your Back Pain*. Ontario, Canada: Backfitpro Inc.

Sahrmann, S. 2002. *Diagnosis and Treatment of Movement Impairment Syndromes*. St. Louis, MO: Mosby.

Schmidt, R.A. 1991. *Motor Learning and Performance: From Principles to Practice*. Champaign, IL: Human Kinetics.

Verstegen, M., and P. Williams. 2004. *Core Performance: The Revolutionary Workout Program to Transform Your Body and Your Life*. New York, NY: Rodale.

Youdas, J.W., B.R. Guck, R.C. Hebrink, J.D. Rugotzke, T.J. Madson, and J.H. Hollman. 2008. "An Electromyographic Analysis of the Ab-Slide Exercise, Abdominal Crunch, Supine Double Leg Thrust, and Side Bridge in Healthy Young Adults: Implications for Rehabilitation Professionals." *Journal of Strength and Conditioning Research* 22(6): 1939-46.

Chapter 4

Bryner R.W., I.H. Ullrich, J. Sauers, D. Donley, G. Hornsby, M. Kolar, and R. Yeater. 1999. "Effects of Resistance Vs. Aerobic Training Combined With an 800 Calorie Liquid Diet on Lean Body Mass and Resting Metabolic Rate." *Journal of the American College of Nutrition* 18(2): 115-121.

Cosgrove, A. 2007. "The Hierarchy of Fat Loss." *T-Nation*, April 11, 2007. www.t-nation.com/training/hierarchy-of-fat-loss.

Demling, R.H., and L. DeSanti. 2000. "Effect of a Hypocaloric Diet, Increased Protein Intake and Resistance Training on Lean Mass Gains and Fat Mass Loss in Overweight Police Officers." *Annals of Nutrition and Metabolism* 44(1): 21-9.

Dolezal, B., J. Potteiger, D. Jacobsen, and S. Benedict. 2000. "Muscle Damage and Resting Metabolic Rate after Acute Resistance Exercise With an Eccentric Overload." *Medicine and Science in Sports and Exercise* 32(7): 1202-7.

Donnelly J.E., T. Sharp, J. Houmard, M.G. Carlson, J.O. Hill, J.E. Whatley, and R.G. Israel. 1993. "Muscle Hypertrophy with Large-Scale Weight Loss and Resistance Training." *American Journal of Clinical Nutrition* 58(4): 561-5.

Elliot, D.L., L. Goldberg, and K.S. Kuehl. 1988. "Does Aerobic Conditioning Cause a Sustained Increase in Metabolic Rate?" *American Journal of Medicine and Science* 296(4): 249-51.

Geliebter, A., M.M. Maher, L. Gerace, B. Gutin, S.B. Heymsfield, and S.A. Hashim. 1997. "Effects of Strength or Aerobic Training on Body Composition, Resting Metabolic Rate, and Peak Oxygen Consumption in Obese Dieting Subjects." *American Journal of Clinical Nutrition* 66(3): 557-63.

Hunter, G.R. et al. 2008. "Resistance Training Conserves Fat-Free Mass and Resting Energy Expenditure Following Weight Loss." *Obesity (Silver Spring)* 16(5): 1045-51.

Hunter, G.R., D.R. Bryan, C.J. Wetzstein, P.A. Zuckerman, and M.M. Bamman. 2002. "Resistance Training and Intra-abdominal Adipose Tissue in Older Men and Women." *Medicine and Science in Sports and Exercise* 34(6): 1023-8.

Hunter, G., G. Fisher, W. Neumeier, S. Carter, and E. Plaisance. 2015. "Exercise Training and Energy Expenditure Following Weight Loss." *Medicine and Science in Sports and Exercise* 47(9): 1950-7.

Hunter, G.R., C.J. Wetzstein, D.A. Fields, A. Brown, and M.M. Bamman. 2000. "Resistance Training Increases Total Energy Expenditure and Free-Living Physical Activity in Older Adults." *Journal of Applied Physiology* 89(3): 977-84.

Kelleher, A.R., K.J. Hackney, T.J. Fairchild, S. Keslacy, and L.L. Ploutz-Snyder. 2010. "The Metabolic Costs of Reciprocal Supersets Vs. Traditional Resistance Exercise in Young Recreationally Active Adults." *Journal of Strength and Conditioning Research* 24(4): 1043-51.

Kraemer, W.J., and J.S. Volek et al. 1999. "Influence of Exercise Training on Physiological and Performance Changes With Weight Loss in Men." *Medicine and Science in Sports and Exercise* 31(9): 1320-9.

Mazzetti, S., et al. 2007. "Effect of Explosive Versus Slow Contractions and Exercise Intensity on Energy Expenditure." *Medicine and Science in Sports and Exercise* 39(8): 1291-301.

Poehlman, E.T., and C. Melby. 1998. "Resistance Training and Energy Balance." *International Journal of Sport Nutrition and Exercise Metabolism* 8(2): 143-59.

"Rate-limiting step." *A Dictionary of Biology. Encyclopedia.com.* (May 19, 2020). https://www.encyclopedia.com/science/dictionaries-thesauruses-pictures-and-press-releases/rate-limiting-step.

Scott, C., M. Leary, and A. Tenbraak. 2011. "Energy Expenditure Characteristics of Weight lifting: 2 Sets to Fatigue. *Applied Physiology, Nutrition, and Metabolism* 36(1): 115-20.

Shiraev, T., and G. Barclay. 2012. "Evidence Based Exercise: Clinical Benefits of High Intensity Interval Training." *Australian Family Physician* 41: 960-2.

Tremblay, A., J.A. Simoneau, and C. Bouchard. 1994. "Impact of Exercise Intensity on Body Fatness and Skeletal Muscle Metabolism." *Metabolism* 43(7): 814-8.

Chapter 5

French, D. 2016. "Adaptations to Anaerobic Training Programs." In *Essentials of Strength Training and Conditioning*, 4th ed., edited by G. Haff, and N.T. Triplett, 87-114. Champaign, IL: Human Kinetics.

Helms, E. , A. Morgan, and A. Valdez. 2019. *The Muscle and Strength Pyramid: Training*. Self-published.

McLester J.R., P. Bishop, and M.E. Guilliams. 2000. "Comparison of 1 Day and 3 Days per Week of Equal-Volume Resistance Training in Experienced Subjects." *Journal of Strength and Conditioning Research* 14: 273-81.

Myers, Thomas W. 2001. *Anatomy Trains: Myofascial Meridians for Manual and Movement Therapists*. Edinburgh: Churchill Livingstone.

Rhea, M. R., S.D. Ball, W.T. Phillips, and L.N. Burkett. 2002. "A Comparison of Linear and Daily Undulating Periodized Programs With Equated Volume and Intensity for Strength." *Journal of Strength and Conditioning Research* 16(2): 250-5.

Schoenfeld, B.J. 2010. "The Mechanisms of Muscle Hypertrophy and Their Application to Resistance Training." *Journal of Strength and Conditioning Research* 24(10): 2857-72.

Schoenfeld, B. 2011. "The Use of Specialized Training Techniques to Maximize Muscle Hypertrophy." *Strength and Conditioning Journal* 33(4): 60-5.

Schoenfeld, B.J., et al., 2014. "Effects of Different Volume-Equated Resistance Training Loading Strategies on Muscular Adaptations in Well-Trained Men." *Journal of Strength and Conditioning Research* 28(10): 2909-18.

Schoenfeld, B.J., et al., 2015. "Influence of Resistance Training Frequency on Muscular Adaptations in Well-Trained Men." *Journal of Strength and Conditioning Research* 29(7): 1821–9.

Schoenfeld, B.J., et al. 2015. "Effects of Low- Versus High-Load Resistance Training on Muscle Strength and Hypertrophy in Well-Trained Men." *Journal of Strength and Conditioning Research* 29(10): 2954-63.

Schoenfeld, B.J., et al., 2016. "Effects of Resistance Training Frequency on Measures of Muscle Hypertrophy: A Systematic Review and Meta-analysis." *Sports Medicine* 46(11): 1689–97.

Schoenfeld B.J., D. Ogborn, and J.W. Krieger. 2017. "Dose-Response Relationship Between Weekly Resistance Training Volume and Increases in Muscle Mass: A Systematic Review and Meta-analysis." *Journal of Sports Sciences* 35(11): 1073-82.

Wernbom, M., J. Augustsson, and R. Thomee. 2007. "The Influence of Frequency, Intensity, Volume and Mode of Strength Training on Whole Muscle Cross-Sectional Area in Humans." *Sports Medicine (Auckland, NZ)* 37: 225-64.

Zourdos, M.C. 2018. "Can You Simply Count the Number of Sets to Quantify Volume?" *Monthly Applications in Strength Sport (MASS)* 2(9). https://www.strongerbyscience.com/mass/

Zourdos, M.C., et al., 2016. "Novel Resistance Training-Specific RPE Scale Measuring Repetitions in Reserve." *Journal of Strength Conditioning Research* 30(1): 267-75.

Chapter 6
Ralston, G.W., L. Kilgore, F.B. Wyatt, J.S. Baker. 2017. "The Effect of Weekly Set Volume on Strength Gain: A Meta-Analysis." *Sports Medicine* 47, 2585-2601. doi:10.1007/s40279-017-0762-7.

Rhea, M.R., et al., 2003. "A Meta-Analysis to Determine the Dose Response for Strength Development." *Medicine and Science in Sports and Exercise* 35(3): 456-64.

Selye, H. 1956. *The Stress of Life*. New York: McGraw-Hill.

Staley, C. 2003. "Periodization That Works." *T-Nation*, May 2, 2003. www.t-nation.com/workouts/periodization-that-works.

Tsatsouline, P. 2003. *The Naked Warrior*. St. Paul, MN: Dragon Door.

"What Is Homeostasis? - Definition & Examples." Study.com. September 3, 2015. https://study.com/academy/lesson/what-is-homeostasis-definition-examples-quiz.html.

Chapter 7
Poliquin, C. 1988. "Five Ways to Increase the Effectiveness of Your Strength Training Program." *NSCA Journal* 10(3): 34-39.

Chapter 9
Cosgrove, A. 2011. "EFS Classic: Your Body Is Barbell: No Dumbbells, No Barbells, No Problem." *Elite FTS*, December 24, 2011. https://www.elitefts.com/education/motivation/your-body-is-a-barbell-no-dumbbells-no-barbells-no-problem/

About the Authors

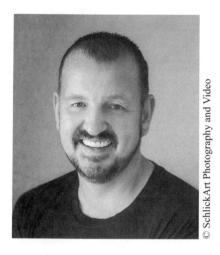

© SchlickArt Photography and Video

Alwyn Cosgrove, CSCS, is co-owner (with his wife, Rachel) of Results Fitness in Santa Clarita, California—twice named one of the top 10 gyms in America by *Men's Health* and *Women's Health* magazines. Alwyn and Rachel are also owners of a fitness professional consulting company, Results Fitness University.

Cosgrove studied sports performance at West Lothian College and then went on to receive a sports science degree with honors from Chester, a college of the University of Liverpool. During his career as a fitness coach, Cosgrove has studied under top fitness professionals and coaches in the world and has worked with a wide variety of clientele, from the general population to top-level athletes and world champions in a multitude of sports.

A nationally known speaker, Cosgrove has coauthored nine best-selling fitness books, is a member of the Nike Performance Council, and has been a presenter on the Perform Better tour for more than a decade.

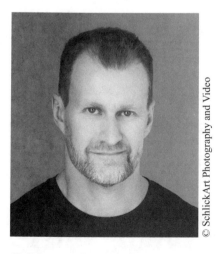

© SchlickArt Photography and Video

Craig Rasmussen, CSCS, is the director of coaching and programming at Results Fitness in Santa Clarita, California. He has more than 18 years of experience in the fitness industry and has worked with all levels, ages, and types of clientele—including professional athletes and general population clients with a wide variety of goals. Previously, he worked as a credentialed physical education teacher at the middle school level in Santa Monica, California.

Rasmussen is certified as a strength and conditioning specialist through the National Strength and Conditioning Association. He received his bachelor of arts degree in physical education from California State University at Chico. With an unquenchable thirst for learning and sharing what he has learned with others, he also holds coaching and programming certifications from several top-level organizations in the fitness industry. He has been featured in numerous magazines, including *Muscle & Fitness*, *Men's Fitness*, *Men's Health*, and *T Nation*.

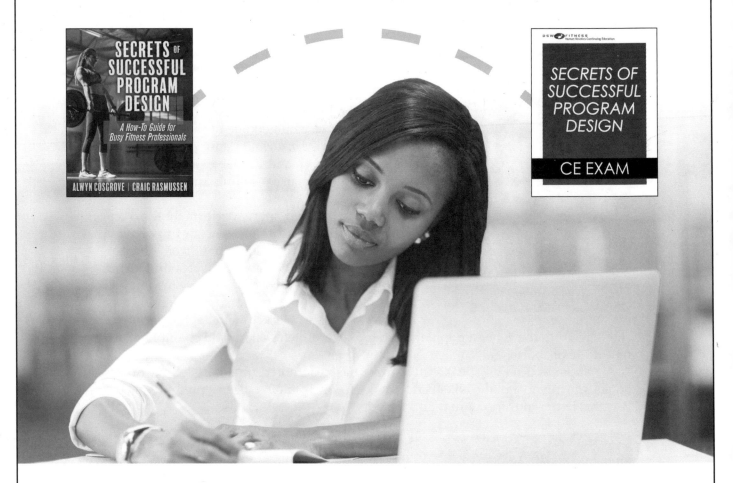
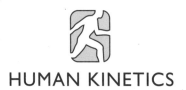